# MCQs for the MRCS
# Examination
## (Applied Basic Sciences with
## Explanatory Answers)

# MCQs for the MRCS Examination
## (Applied Basic Sciences with Explanatory Answers)

**Rahij Anwar**

MBBS MS (Ortho) [India]

MSc (Trauma) MRCS (Ed) [United Kingdom]

Honorary Fellow of Institute of Accident Surgery, Birmingham, UK

Registrar

Trauma and Orthopaedics

The Royal London Hospital

United Kingdom

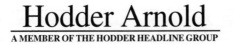

Hodder Arnold

A MEMBER OF THE HODDER HEADLINE GROUP

First published in India in 2004 by Jaypee Brothers, Medical Publishers (P) Ltd,
EMCA House, 23/23B Ansari Road, Daryaganj, New Delhi 110 002, India

First published in the United Kingdom in 2005 by Hodder Arnold,
an imprint of Hodder Education and a member of the Hodder Headline Group,
338 Euston Road, London NW1 3BH

**http://www.hoddereducation.co.uk**

This UK edition distributed in the United States of America by
Oxford University Press Inc.,
198 Madison Avenue, New York, NY10016
Oxford is a registered trademark of Oxford University Press

Whilst the advice and information in this book are believed to be true and accurate
at the date of going to press, neither the author[s] nor the publisher can accept any
legal responsibility or liability for any errors or omissions that may be made. In
particular (but without limiting the generality of the preceding disclaimer) every
effort has been made to check drug dosages; however it is still possible that errors
have been missed. Furthermore, dosage schedules are constantly being revised and
new side-effects recognized. For these reasons the reader is strongly urged to consult
the drug companies' printed instructions before administering any of the drugs
recommended in this book.

*British Library Cataloguing in Publication Data*
A catalogue record for this book is available from the British Library

*Library of Congress Cataloging-in-Publication Data*
A catalog record for this book is available from the Library of Congress

ISBN-10 [normal]    0 340 90583 2
ISBN-13             978 0 340 90583 8

1 2 3 4 5 6 7 8 9 10

Cover Designer:    Nichola Smith

*Typeset at* JPBMP typesetting unit
*Printed at* Replika Press Pvt. Ltd. Kundli 131 028

What do you think about this book? Or any other Hodder Arnold title?
Please send your comments to www.hoddereducation.co.uk

Dedicated to

**The Late Syed Zakiul Hasan Zaidi, a Professor of Botany**

*Who conducted free coaching classes at his home to help the students pass the highly competitive MBBS entrance exams. These classes were open to all the serious students and continued throughout the year. The heat was sweltering and temperature reached 40 degrees Celsius; there were frequent power failures. When once asked why the coaching was provided for nothing, his answer was, "I am just trying to repay my own teachers, who funded my education throughout my career". What a noble repayment!*

*Many students successfully passed the entrance exam and became doctors, due at least in part to his untiring efforts, and I was one of them. Unfortunately, he died prematurely in 1990, whilst undergoing surgery. He will be remembered for his wealth of knowledge, dedication and high moral values by many generations to come.*

*and*

**The Teachers of Our Lady of Fatima School, Aligarh**

*Who laid the foundation of my interest in literature*

# Foreword

Comprehensive coverage for surgical examinations is all important and the curriculum for basic surgical tests, such as the Membership for the Royal College of Surgeons requires a sound and accurate knowledge of all aspects of surgical care.

This textbook of multiple choice questions covers the spectrum for revision in surgery and provides a stimulus to understanding many of the aspects of surgical diagnosis and preoperative planning, and perioperative care required as preparation. This book achieves a good balance in providing the necessary impetus to reading and research for general knowledge in all aspects of surgery. It is set out in an accurate and easily read form, and will be an invaluable adjunct to study for the primary exam in surgery. Self-assessment with this book is highly recommended in preparation for the MRCS examination.

**TM Bucknill** RD, MBBS, FRCS,
Consultant Trauma and Orthopaedic Surgeon
Bart's and the London NHS Trust
Regional Speciality Advisor in Orthopaedics
London Deanery and North-East Thames

# Foreword

# *Preface*

The examination system of the Royal Colleges of Surgery has undergone major changes in the last few years. The former 'FRCS' has now been renamed as 'MRCS' and the knowledge required has changed considerably. The membership exam places emphasis on the identification and management of surgical emergencies and common conditions. Attention is focussed on the understanding of basic concepts related to surgical conditions; the exam deliberately avoids the minute details of diseases and operations, which trainees will learn at a later stage. The new exam is, in many ways, simpler than the old FRCS, but nevertheless it does cover the entirety of surgery and aims to test the breadth of knowledge.

This book, like any other MCQs book, should not be regarded as a substitute for the textbooks which every student should read before in preparation for an attempt at the exam. The multiple choice questions will test and educate the readers. However, I have carefully selected those topics that frequently appear in the examinations. I have compiled the questions based on the syllabus of the examination and for simplicity, provided the answers on the same page. At the end of each chapter more details are available. I hope this format will save precious time.

The book is divided into various sections based on the syllabuses of the Royal Colleges. I have tried to cover all the important topics that appear frequently in the exams. There are some topics which are covered in more depth. This indicates that the reader is expected to have a more thorough knowledge of these important topics. It does not, however, mean that those topics that are less well represented are unimportant. This includes not only the surgical conditions but also subjects like medical emergencies, audit, medicolegal problems, and theatre design.

I recommend that you attempt the MCQs in this book once you have studied properly, and feel yourself confident enough to answer the questions. Students may prefer attempting the questions first and then going back to the textbook to read in detail. I have no objections, but remember that all topics may not be covered and you may end up being a loser! However, for a few this MCQs book might become a driving force for further reading. No matter what approach you adopt, avoid doing the test papers until you find yourself completely ready for the exam.

Good luck!

**Rahij Anwar**

# *Acknowledgements*

I slept and dreamt that life was joy
I awoke and saw that life was service
I acted and behold, service was joy
—Rabindranath Tagore

I am extremely grateful to Mr RP Mackenney, Dr AM Khan, Mr H Fareed and Mr Jagjeevanram for their valuable contributions in the advancement of my career.

Dr Zafar Iqbal, who has a special interest in literature, Mr S Neshat Anjum and all other friends provided immense support and encouragement in the completion of this book. I am also grateful to Dr Nitish Gogi for designing the cover page by using his excellent IT skills.

I wish to thank Mr TM Bucknill, Miss Swee Ang and all other members of the Department of Orthopaedics at the Royal London Hospital for their guidance and co-operation.

I am indeed very grateful to Mr Simon Owen-Johnstone for making valuable suggestions to improve the general outline of the book.

This work would never have been completed without the untiring efforts of my wife, Huma, who provided constant help and moral support. She made special efforts in finding an excellent Secretary, Ms Teresa Trotman, for typing the manuscript.

I am particularly grateful to Mr JP Vij, Chairman and Managing Director and Mr Tarun Duneja, General Manager (Publishing), Jaypee Brothers Medical Publishers (P) Ltd. for their patience. I would like to acknowledge the help of The Royal College of

Surgeons of Edinburgh and JN Medical College, Aligarh in providing the photograph for the cover page.

Last, but not least, I wish to express my gratitude to my teachers at Our Lady of Fatima School and at JN Medical College, AMU, Aligarh, India; these people shaped my personality and played a significant role in the development of my interest in surgery and literature.

# Contents

# 1

## Perioperative Management

1. **A patient with Type I diabetes, having a major elective surgery should ideally:**
   A. Receive a single dose of preoperative short acting insulin and then normal dose postoperatively
   B. Be prioritised on the operation list
   C. Get no insulin during surgery
   D. Have IV insulin through an insulin pump in the perioperative period
   E. Be starved for much longer than the normal patients

2. **Smoking causes:**
   A. A shift of the oxygen-dissociation curve to the right
   B. A reduction in the heart rate and systemic arterial blood pressure
   C. No change in the cardiovascular function when stopped 12-24 hours before surgery
   D. Impairment of the wound healing and immune function
   E. Increase in the oxygen demand

3. **In patients with chronic obstructive airway disease (COAD):**
   A. The risk of postoperative respiratory failure is decreased if $FEV_1/FVC$ ratio is less than 50%
   B. Arterial blood gas analysis is not required preoperatively if the oxygen saturation is 89% and the chest X-ray is normal
   C. Hypoxia in the postoperative period is never due to inadequate ventilation or respiratory depression with opiates
   D. Chest physiotherapy, stopping smoking and adequate pain relief promotes good respiratory function, postoperatively
   E. Preoperative baseline lung function tests are necessary

---

1. A:F, B:T, C:F, D:T, E:F        2. A:F, B:F, C:F, D:T, E:T
3. A:F, B:F, C:F, D:T, E:T

4. **Jaundiced patients undergoing surgery:**
   A. Should be well hydrated
   B. Should have a preoperative clotting screen, especially the prothrombin time
   C. Should receive prophylactic antibiotics in the presence of a biliary obstruction
   D. May have compromised respiratory and renal functions
   E. May require vitamin K and fresh frozen plasma

5. **A 72 years old patient who was due to have a total knee replacement develops a massive MI twelve hours before his surgery. The surgery was cancelled because of the following reason (s):**
   A. The risk of re-infarction is more than 75% in the first three weeks following an MI
   B. The rehabilitation from the operation would be delayed
   C. The chances of postoperative infection were high
   D. To avoid a detailed anaesthetic and cardiovascular assessment
   E. It was safer to perform the operation four weeks following the MI

6. **The major risk factors for Deep Vein Thrombosis are:**
   A. Early postoperative mobilisation
   B. Age
   C. Pregnancy
   D. Oral contraceptive drugs
   E. Malignancy

7. **The following features are characteristic of DVT:**
   A. Seen in ~30% of surgical patients
   B. Sixty-five percent of below knee DVTs are asymptomatic
   C. Calf tenderness and swelling are quite common
   D. Can be confused with a ruptured Baker's cyst
   E. Duplex ultrasound and venogram aid in diagnosis

---

4. A:T, B:T, C:T, D:T, E:T          5. A:T, B:F, C:F, D:F, E:F
6. A:F, B:T, C:T, D:T, E:T          7. A:T, B:T, C:T, D:T, E:T

8. **DVT can be prevented by:**
   A. The use of graduated compression stockings
   B. Applying pneumatic foot pumps during surgery
   C. A course of contraceptive pills and hormonal replacement therapy
   D. Early postoperative mobilisation
   E. The use of tourniquet during the operation

9. **Virchow's triad:**
   A. Describes changes in the supraclavicular lymph node
   B. Describes factors leading to the deep vein thrombosis
   C. Consists of endothelial damage, hypercoagulability and sluggish blood blow
   D. Also explains changes in the wall of the heart in IHD
   E. Suggests prognosis in Ca stomach

10. **Steroids:**
    A. Promote wound healing
    B. Are contraindicated in patients with Crohn's disease having surgery under general anaesthesia
    C. Cause skin and musculoskeletal changes
    D. Cause water depletion and sodium retention
    E. Can be used in the perioperative period for endocrinal abnormalities

11. **Sickle cell anaemia:**
    A. Can precipitate a crisis during surgery
    B. Is common in people of Caucasian origin
    C. Causes increased susceptibility to infection
    D. Crisis can be prevented by adequate hydration and avoiding hypoxia
    E. Involves the replacement of Hb A by Hb F

8. A:T, B:T, C:F, D:T, E:F          9.  A:F, B:T, C:T, D:F, E:F
10. A:F, B:F, C:T, D:F, E:T          11. A:T, B:F, C:T, D:T, E:F

**6** 📄 **MCQs for the MRCS Examination**

12. **Informed consent:**
    A. Involves explanation of the treatment, options available and possible risks and benefits to the patient
    B. Can be signed by a close relative of the patient
    C. Should preferably be taken by the operating surgeon
    D. Is invalid if taken after the administration of midazolam
    E. Can be taken from a child 10 years of age

13. **Pulse oximetry:**
    A. Is an invasive method for continuous measure of oxygen saturation in the arterial blood
    B. Actually measures the partial pressure of oxygen
    C. A value of 98% suggests adequate peripheral oxygenation
    D. Is not affected by the levels of carboxyhaemoglobin in the blood
    E. Is not reliable in the presence of profound anaemia and hypothermia

14. **Malignant hyperthermia:**
    A. Is a common condition affecting surgical patients of Caucasian origin
    B. Is a familial X-linked disorder
    C. IV Dantrolene sodium and supportive measures help to control the condition
    D. Is characterised by a rise in the temperature and acidosis due to rigidity
    E. Can lead to renal failure

15. **Premedication is prescribed preoperatively for:**
    A. Reducing bleeding during surgery
    B. Allaying anxiety
    C. Drying secretions
    D. Analgesia
    E. Regional anaesthesia only

---

12. A:T, B:F, C:T, D:T, E:F        13. A:F, B:F, C:T, D:F, E:T
14. A:F, B:F, C:T, D:T, E:T        15. A:F, B:T, C:T, D:T, E:F

16. **Non–depolarising muscle relaxants:**
    A. Common example is suxamethonium
    B. Are competitive inhibitors of acetylcholine receptors on muscle-end plates
    C. Time of onset is 15-20 minutes
    D. Have intrinsic anaesthetic effect
    E. Atracurium and vecuronium should never be used as infusions

17. **Tourniquet:**
    A. Can cause neurovascular complications
    B. Reperfusion period can exceed to 180 minutes for the lower limb from the time of application
    C. Can precipitate a sickle cell crisis
    D. Cuff pressure should be set at 50 mmHg and 100 mmHg above the systolic pressure in the upper and lower limbs, respectively
    E. Should not be used for finger surgery

18. **Suxamethonium is known to cause:**
    A. Depolarisation and is very suitable for crash induction
    B. Tachycardia in children
    C. Hypokalaemia by preventing release of potassium from muscle cells
    D. Scoline apnoea
    E. Malignant hyperthermia

19. **Lignocaine:**
    A. Acts by inducing a blockade of nerve transmission in peripheral nerve impulses
    B. Has toxic central nervous and cardiovascular effects
    C. Maximum safe dose is 15 mg/kg
    D. Maximum safe dose with adrenaline is 5 mg/kg
    E. Is safe to use with adrenaline near end arteries (e.g. digits, penis)

---

16. A:F, B:T, C:F, D:F, E:F      17. A:T, B:F, C:T, D:T, E:F
18. A:T, B:F, C:F, D:T, E:T      19. A:T, B:T, C:F, D:T, E:F

20. **Bupivacaine:**
    A. Can't be used for epidural blocks and postoperative wound infiltration
    B. Unlike lignocaine has no cardiovascular toxic effects
    C. Safe dose is 3mg/kg with and 2mg/kg without adrenaline
    D. Has a much shorter action than lignocaine
    E. Can be used for spinal anaesthesia

21. **Central venous pressure:**
    A. Represents the right atrial pressure
    B. Normal value is 10-15 mmHg
    C. Catheter introduction can cause infection, haemorrhage and pneumothorax
    D. Line should not be used for administration of parenteral nutrition
    E. Catheter is preferably inserted through the right external jugular vein and the tip should float in the left atrium

22. **Pulmonary artery catheter:**
    A. Measures the left atrial pressure reasonably accurately
    B. Can be used to measure the cardiac output by thermodilution
    C. Is not indicated in patients with a complicated cardiac history undergoing complex surgical operations
    D. Useful in patients with a multisystem failure
    E. Is multiluminal and the normal pulmonary artery pressure is 6-12 mmHg

23. **Diathermy:**
    A. Involves the passage of a low frequency direct current (DC) through the body tissues
    B. High local temperatures of upto 1000 °C may be produced
    C. Monopolar generates lower power than bipolar
    D. A patient electrode is essential in the bipolar type
    E. Bipolar is useful for surgery of penis or on digits

---

20. A:F, B:F, C:T, D:F, E:T      21. A:T, B:F, C:T, D:F, E:F
22. A:T, B:T, C:F, D:T, E:T      23. A:F, B:T, C:F, D:F, E:T

24. **Sterilization:**
    A. By ethylene oxide is not suitable for rubber or plastic
    B. Is the same as disinfection but the reduction in the number of microorganism is higher in the latter
    C. By gamma radiation is very useful for catheters and syringes
    D. By steam under pressure involves the use of an autoclave
    E. By formaldehyde is not suitable for heat sensitive equipment

25. A 66 years old patient develops severe retrosternal pain after supper, three days following a total hip replacement. The pain, sharp in nature, radiated to the interscapular region. He also has nausea but no vomiting. He is a known hypertensive and a chronic smoker. On examination, he is found to be normotensive, tachycardic with a pulse rate of 105/min and tachypnoeic. Few basal crackles are heard on chest auscultation, on both sides. The radiograph of the chest is normal. Full blood count, urea and electrolytes, blood gases and cardiac enzymes performed within few minutes of the onset of pain are all within normal limits. ECG taken 5 minutes after the onset of pain demonstrates tachycardia but no significant ST elevation or T-inversion:
    A. Pulmonary embolism is the most likely diagnosis
    B. This patient should have an urgent V/Q scan
    C. High flow oxygen and pain relief are essential
    D. High-dose anticoagulation should be commenced immediately
    E. Cardiac enzymes, arterial blood gases and ECG should be repeated after 24 hours

26. Postoperative pyrexia:
    A. Within 24 hours after a large bowel resection suggests a wound infection
    B. Within 48 hours of surgery with cough and a radiopaque shadow on the lung is suggestive of a chest infection
    C. After 24 hours should be investigated thoroughly
    D. Appearing in a relatively healthy looking but immobile patient with some leg swelling suggests pulmonary embolism
    E. Occurring due to a wound infection or an anastomotic leak is usually seen 2 weeks after surgery

27. A sixty-nine years old obese hypertensive lady, who has been on HRT for sometime, undergoes a successful operation for a colonic carcinoma. She develops acute shortness of breath on the fifth day of the operation. On examination, she is hypotensive, tachypnoeic and anxious. Her oxygen saturation falls to 83% on air but returns to normal on 100% oxygen. Chest X-ray shows some cardiomegaly and a very small radiopaque shadow in the left lung. Her arterial blood gases demonstrate hypoxia and acidosis. ECG reveals sinus tachycardia:
    A. The most likely diagnosis is secondaries in the lung
    B. Anticoagulation should be considered
    C. A CT scan of the chest should be requested on an urgent basis
    D. Close monitoring and frequent arterial blood gas sampling may be necessary
    E. Radiotherapy and chemotherapy may become necessary due to the present complication

---

26. A:F, B:T, C:T, D:F, E:F        27.  A:F, B:T, C:F, D:T, E:F

28. **Blood transfusion can cause:**
    A. Hypokalaemia
    B. A shift of the oxyhaemoglobin curve to the right
    C. Transmission of infections
    D. Coagulation abnormalities
    E. Immunological reactions

29. **Non-steroidal anti-inflammatory drugs:**
    A. Can be safely given in the presence of renal failure
    B. Provide a sustained postoperative analgesia when given through a pump
    C. Should be avoided in patients with a history of peptic ulceration and bronchial asthma
    D. Act on $\mu/\kappa/\Delta$ receptors
    E. Are known to interact with warfarin

30. **Postoperative hypoxaemia:**
    A. Can be regarded as a $PaO_2$ less than 13kPa (60 mmHg)
    B. Is an important cause of confusion in the elderly
    C. Initially causes a gradual fall in ventilation
    D. Causes tachycardia and this may result in myocardial ischaemia
    E. Has no relation to wound healing

31. **Carboxyhaemoglobin:**
    A. Levels in blood are relatively high in smokers
    B. Accelerates binding of haemoglobin to oxygen
    C. Levels of upto 15% in heavy smokers can be reversed by stopping smoking even for 24 hours
    D. Has no effects on the cardiovascular system
    E. Inhibits the ability of Hb to give up oxygen

32. **Arterial blood gas analysis:**
    A. Can give a relatively accurate assessment of partial pressure of oxygen in the blood
    B. Does not change with temperature
    C. Should never be carried out in a heparinised sample
    D. Is ineffective in the diagnosis of metabolic acidosis
    E. Should be done soon after taking a sample

28. A:F, B:F, C:T, D:T, E:T    29. A:F, B:F, C:T, D:F, E:T
30. A:F, B:T, C:F, D:T, E:F    31. A:T, B:F, C:T, D:F, E:T
32. A:T, B:F, C:F, D:F, E:T

33. **Oxygen delivery is:**
    A. A product of stroke volume and oxygen content
    B. Determined by the oxygen saturation
    C. Affected by trauma, exercise, surgery or infection
    D. Not increased by an increase in the cardiac output
    E. About 200 ml/minute at rest

34. **Postoperative hypotension can be caused by:**
    A. Drugs
    B. Haemorrhage
    C. Septicaemia
    D. Deep vein thrombosis
    E. Myocardial infarction

35. **Pulmonary embolism may cause:**
    A. Severe chest pain
    B. Shortness of breath
    C. Hypertension
    D. Haemoptysis
    E. SI QIII TIII pattern in the ECG

36. **Commonly used absorbable sutures in surgical practice are:**
    A. Polypropylene
    B. Polyamide
    C. Polydiaxonone
    D. Polyglactin
    E. Polyester

37. **The following are known to cause bleeding tendencies:**
    A. Liver disorders
    B. Warfarin
    C. Diazepam
    D. DIC
    E. Factor VIII deficiency

---

33. A:F, B:T, C:T, D:F, E:F    34. A:T, B:T, C:T, D:F, E:T
35. A:T, B:T, C:F, D:T, E:T    36. A:F, B:F, C:T, D:T, E:F
37. A:T, B:T, C:F, D:T, E:T

**38. Keloid scars are:**
   A. Limited to the boundaries of the original wound
   B. Formed by abnormal fat metabolism
   C. More common in Caucasians
   D. Commonly seen over sternum, shoulder and extensor surfaces
   E. A common sequelae of wound infection

**39. pH:**
   A. Is defined as the negative logarithm of hydrogen ion concentration
   B. Of more than 7.44 indicates acidaemia
   C. Has no relation to bicarbonate:carbonic acid ratio
   D. Normal range is 7.44–7.64
   E. Is increased in conditions which cause alkalosis

**40. The following are normal values for an adult patient:**
   A. pH 7.36-7.44
   B. $PO_2$ 10-14 kPa (75-100 mmHg)
   C. $PCO_2$ 2-4 kPa (17-35 mmHg)
   D. Standard bicarbonate 15-17 mmol/l
   E. Base excess −2 to +2

**41. Normal adult daily requirement of:**
   A. Water is 15 ml per kg body weight
   B. Na, K and Cl, each, is approx 1mmol/kg body weight
   C. $Ca^{2+}$ is 1 mol/kg body weight
   D. $Mg^{2+}$ is 7 mmol
   E. Phosphate is 14 mmol

**42. Metabolic response to surgery (injury) causes the following renal effects:**
   A. Increase in the GFR
   B. Enhanced tubular reabsorption of sodium ions
   C. Increased water loss due to a fall in ADH production
   D. Vasodilatation due to pain and blood loss
   E. Protein catabolism

43. **Distribution of the total body water in a 70 kg man is as follows:**
    A. ¼ extracellular and ¾ intracellular
    B. Plasma contributes 3.5 l and is in extracelluar compartment
    C. 8.5 litres is in the intracellular compartment
    D. Total extracellular fluid is about 15 litres
    E. Total interstitial fluid (tissue fluid) is 2.8 litres

44. **Hartmann's solution:**
    A. Is also known as Ringer's lactate
    B. Contains 131 mmol/l of sodium ions
    C. Has no potassium
    D. Should be avoided in the perioperative period
    E. Contains higher sodium ion content than the normal saline

45. **Hypokalaemia:**
    A. Can be precipitated by the use of diuretics
    B. May occur in Crohn's disease
    C. Presents as muscle weakness, hypotonia and cardiac arrythmias
    D. May be a feature in intestinal obstruction
    E. Can be be corrected by a rapid injection of potassium as a bolus

46. **In vitamin K deficiency:**
    A. PT and APTT are always normal
    B. Platelet count is markedly low
    C. TT is normal
    D. Synthesis of Factors II, VII, IX and X is affected
    E. Bleeding is rarely a problem

47. **Prostaglandins:**
    A. Cause vasoconstriction and platelet segregation
    B. Are produced mainly by lymphocytes
    C. Are produced by the lipoxygenase pathway
    D. Are inhibited by aspirin
    E. Cannot cause leucocytosis and a raised temperature

---

43. A:F, B:T, C:F, D:T, E:F      44. A:T, B:T, C:F, D:F, E:F
45. A:T, B:T, C:T, D:T, E:F      46. A:F, B:F, C:T, D:T, E:F
47. A:F, B:F, C:F, D:T, E:F

48. **Tumour necrosis factor alpha (TNF α):**
    A. Is also known as cachectin
    B. Is one of the main cytokines
    C. Has a potential to cause multiple organ dysfunction syndrome
    D. Released from basophils
    E. Inhibits the production of other cytokines and APRs

49. **Interferons:**
    A. Are produced by the T lymphocytes, leucocytes and fibroblasts
    B. Inhibit viral replication
    C. Especially γ interferon, accelerate prostaglandins release
    D. Enhance MHC expression
    E. Improve cytotoxicity against certain target cancer cells

50. **The following is true about interleukin-6:**
    A. Is produced by neutrophils only
    B. Has action on immune and haemopoetic systems
    C. Blocks the growth of B-cells
    D. Is not a cytokine
    E. Has an effect on the growth of malignant plasma cells

51. **Type IV hypersensitivity reactions:**
    A. Are typically seen in hay fever
    B. Involve IgE
    C. Provide cell mediated or delayed immunity
    D. Are important in transplant rejections and Mantoux test
    E. Cause release of the mediators from mast cells and basophils

48. A:T, B:T, C:T, D:F, E:F     49. A:T, B:T, C:F, D:T, E:T
50. A:F, B:T, C:F, D:F, E:T     51. A:F, B:F, C:T, D:T, E:F

52. **Wound healing:**
    A. By secondary intervention is seen where the edges of the wound are in close apposition
    B. Is not affected by Transforming growth factor alpha and beta (TGF-α and β)
    C. Is affected significantly by the cytokines, interleukin-1 and Tumour necrosis factor-α
    D. Is delayed with the deficiency of vit C and Zn
    E. Can be stimulated by the administration of steroids

53. **Surgical wounds:**
    A. Can be classified as contaminated or Class III when the rate of infection is about 20%
    B. May dehisce in the presence of infection
    C. Contract by the action of cells called myofibroblasts
    D. Which are badly contaminated can be closed safely provided a proper antibiotic cover is available
    E. Undergo epithelialization, contraction and connective tissue formation

54. **Wound dehiscence:**
    A. May become evident by the discharge of a 'pink fluid' from the postoperative wound after 2-3 days
    B. Does not usually require a second surgery
    C. May prove to be fatal in the absence of a suitable intervention
    D. Occurs more frequently in obese individuals with postoperative cough
    E. Involves partial or total disruption of any or all the layers of the operative wound

55. **Total parenteral nutrition:**
    A. Leads to bacterial translocation from the gut
    B. Is a preferred option in all patients with major intra-abdominal surgery
    C. Is associated with a fatty liver
    D. May cause fluid overload and deficiency or excess of sodium
    E. Rarely requires monitoring of vitamin $B_{12}$/Zinc/Magnesium

---

52. A:F, B:F, C:T, D:T, E:F      53. A:T, B:T, C:T, D:F, E:T
54. A:T, B:F, C:T, D:T, E:T      55. A:T, B:F, C:T, D:T, E:F

56. **Gastric atony can be caused by:**
   A. Ventilation/critical illness
   B. Hyperthyroidism
   C. Head injury
   D. Abdominal surgery
   E. Diabetic neuropathy

57. **Nutritional support:**
   A. May be considered in a preoperative patient with more than 10% weight loss
   B. Is indicated when serum albumin is more than 30 g/l
   C. Through enteral route can cause pulmonary aspiration
   D. Through parenteral route can cause pneumothorax
   E. By parenteral route is safer and doesn't require close monitoring

58. **Principles of management of an abdominal wound dehiscence:**
   A. Resuscitation
   B. Re-exploration
   C. Resuturing
   D. Tight suturing under tension
   E. Peritoneal lavage contraindicated

59. **Features of sepsis:**
   A. Fever or hypothermia
   B. Leucocytosis or leucopenia
   C. Increased urine output
   D. Mental functions never affected
   D. Blood cultures may never be sterile

60. **Helicobacter pylori is associated with:**
   A. Duodenal ulcer
   B. Gastric ulcer
   C. Septic arthritis
   D. Type B antral gastritis
   E. Cellulitis

56. A:T, B:F, C:T, D:T, E:T   57. A:T, B:F, C:T, D:T, E:F
58. A:T, B:T, C:T, D:F, E:F   59. A:T, B:T, C:F, D:F, E:F
60. A:T, B:T, C:F, D:T, E:F

61. **Helicobacter pylori:**
    A. Hydrolyses urea
    B. Can be detected by CLO Test
    C. Always causes gastric acid hyposecretion
    D. May be responsible for hypergastrinaemia in peptic ulcer disease
    E. Has a significantly high recurrence rate following treatment with the triple regimen

62. **Gram-negative organisms are important in:**
    A. Septic shock        B. Tetanus
    C. Cellulitis          D. Gas gangrene
    E. Gastrointestinal infections

63. **Bacteria:**
    A. Osteomyelitis of tibia in a child 3 years of age
    B. Subacute endocarditis after a dental procedure
    C. Perforation of an ulcer preceded by high temp and diarrhoea with a positive blood culture in a developing country
    D. Muscle spasms following a leg laceration in a farming accident
    E. Fluctuant and tender swelling in the left axilla in a 35 years old patient

    1. *Streptococcus viridans*
    2. *H. influenzae*
    3. Salmonella
    4. Clostridium
    5. Neisseria
    6. *E. coli*
    7. *Staphylococcus aureus*
    8. Bacteroides

64. **Exotoxin:**
    A. Classically produced by gram-negative bacteria
    B. Present in the cell wall as a lipopolysaccharide
    C. Common example is tetanoplasmin
    D. Has strong antigenicity
    E. Is heat labile

61. A:T, B:T, C:F, D:T, E:F       62. A:T, B:F, C:F, D:F, E:T
63. A:2, B:1, C:3, D:4, E:8       64. A:F, B:F, C:T, D:T, E:T

65. **Cefuroxime:**
    A. Is a commonly used drug in surgical prophylaxis
    B. 75 % of patients allergic to pencillin are also hypersensitive to cefuroxime
    C. Is a sulphonamide
    D. Has no action against gram-negative organisms
    E. Is contraindicated in joint replacement surgery

66. **The following statements are true about Gas Gangrene:**
    A. Characteristically cause rigidity and muscle spasms
    B. Clostridium perfringens is the causative organism in a majority of the cases
    C. Tetanoplasmin is the exotoxin
    D. Crepitus can usually be detected
    E. Muscle and overlying skin usually normal

67. **MRSA infections:**
    A. Respond well to penicillin and erythromycin
    B. Require barrier nursing
    C. May be screened by taking swabs from the patient and staff
    D. Are not seen in ITU patients
    E. Are difficult to treat

68. **Systemic inflammatory response syndrome consists of:**
    A. Hyperthermia > 38°C
    B. Tachycardia >90/min
    C. White cell count >12 or < 4 × $10^9$/litre
    D. Hypothermia <36°C
    E. None of the above

69. **Patients undergoing primary total hip replacement should:**
    A. Be catheterised preoperatively, on a routine basis
    B. Receive three doses of a broad spectrum antibiotic as prophylaxis
    C. Ideally have no known focus of infection
    D. Proceed to their operation if the urine shows > $10^5$ organisms/ml
    E. Be operated in a theatre with laminar air flow

65. A:T, B:F, C:F, D:F, E:F          66. A:F, B:T, C:F, D:T, E:F
67. A:F, B:T, C:T, D:F, E:T          68. A:T, B:T, C:T, D:T, E:F
69. A:F, B:T, C:T, D:F, E:T

70. **Risk to the surgeons operating on HIV patients can be minimised by:**
    A. 'Double gloving'
    B. Avoiding direct handling of sharp instruments
    C. Using more than normal number of assistants
    D. Preoperative identification of high-risk patients such as homosexuals, IV drug abusers, etc
    E. Haemostasis and avoiding rapid bleeding

71. **Necrotising fasciitis:**
    A. Is always monomicrobial
    B. Involves mainly the skin, subcutaneous tissue and the deep fascia
    C. Patient may require resuscitation
    D. Surgery should be avoided as far as possible
    E. Has a high mortality

72. **Pathogens:**

    A. 34 years old man with a swollen, red and hot right hand and an ascending lymphangitis after an insect bite

    B. Carbuncle in the neck in a patient with Type I diabetes

    C. Kaposi's sarcoma in anal canal

    D. A genetically engineered vaccine is available against it with three initial doses and a booster at five years. Highly recommended to surgeons

    E. Produces antibiotic associated diarrhoea followed by sloughing of the colonic mucosa

    1. *Clostridium difficile*
    2. *Streptococcus pyogenes*
    3. *Mycobacterium tuberculosis*
    4. HPV
    5. *Staphylococcus aureus*
    6. *Hepatitis B virus*
    7. HIV

---

70. A:T, B:T, C:F, D:T, E:T     71. A:F, B:T, C:T, D:F, E:T
72. A:2, B:5, C:7, D:6, E:1

## *Answers*

1. **A:F, B:T, C:F, D:T, E:F**
   Surgery causes an increase in the basal metabolic rate and protein breakdown. This metabolic derangement is more pronounced in diabetics. Neuropathy and cardiovascular dysfunction due to diabetes increase the risk of sudden changes of the arterial blood pressure in the perioperative period. A good diabetic control is essential for a successful outcome. All type I diabetics undergoing major surgery should be given intravenous insulin (sliding scale) during surgery and until eating normally, postoperatively. The diet controlled diabetics and patients on oral agents may also require intravenous insulin sliding scale regimen, if the blood glucose is unstable. Inability to control the blood glucose in the perioperative period can cause ketosis, acidaemia, electrolyte abnormalities and volume depletion. Impairement in wound healing and a diminished immune response may also be seen. It is advisable to put the diabetics first on the operating list to reduce the risk of complications.

2. **A:F, B:F, C:F, D:T, E:T**
   Smoking has a deleterious effect on the outcome of surgery. It influences cardiac, respiratory and immune systems. The carboxyhaemoglobin present in smokers decreases the amount of haemoglobin available for oxygenation and inhibits the ability of haemoglobin to give up oxygen. In other words, the oxygen dissociation curve shifts to the left in smokers.
   Nicotine affects the cardiovascular system by increasing the heart rate and systemic arterial blood pressure. Hence, the supply of oxygen is significantly decreased in smokers with ischaemic heart disease. A significant improvement in the cardiovascular function is expected, if smoking is stopped at least 12 to 24 hours before surgery. Similarly, the respiratory and immune functions may also improve with cessation of smoking at least 6 weeks before surgery.

3. **A:F, B:F, C:F, D:T, E:T**

   Asthma and chronic obstructive airways disease cause generalised airflow obstruction. A thorough assessment is necessary. Spirometry, arterial blood gases, sputum cultures and chest X-ray are important parameters in assessment of the respiratory function. The risk of postoperative respiratory failure is markedly increased if the $FEV_1/FVC$ ratio is less than 50%.

   Nitrous oxide causes tension pneumothorax by rupturing the bullae. Postoperative measures like avoiding smoking, promotion of effective oxygenation, adequate pain relief and chest physiotherapy can improve the respiratory function, dramatically. All infective exacerbations should be treated before surgery.

   Opiates can cause respiratory depression and inadequate ventilation in the perioperative period. Regional anaesthesia has appropriate advantages in respiratory disease.

4. **A:T, B:T, C:T, D:T, E:T**

   Patients with obstructive jaundice are particularly prone to develop renal failure after surgery (hepatorenal syndrome) due to the toxic effects of bilirubin on the kidney. The hepatocellular dysfunction also causes clotting factor deficiencies which results in bleeding disorders.

   A good renal output should be maintained throughout surgery in order to avoid renal failure. This can be achieved by the administration of intravenous fluids and osmotic diuretics. The prothrombin time, if abnormal, should be corrected by the administration of vitamin K or fresh frozen plasma, if required. Prophylactic antibiotics should be advised to avoid cholangitis. Hypoalbuminaemia increases the risk of 'fluid-overload' in such patients. Therefore, close monitoring is essential. Wound failure, infection, renal failure and respiratory compromise are important complications seen in jaundiced patients following surgery.

5. **A:T, B:F, C:F, D:F, E:F**

   Total knee replacement is done on an elective basis. The operation in this patient was cancelled because the risk of re-infarction after a MI is 75% and the mortality due to postoperative MI is quite high. It is safer to cancel the operation for at least 6 months when the mortality or re-infarction rate falls to less than 5%. This patient needs to have a complete anaesthetic and cardiovascular assessment for optimisation of the cardiac status when surgery is contemplated, in future.

   Any surgery in the immediate post-MI period carries a high complication rate and mortality and is best avoided.

6. **A:F, B:T, C:T, D:T, E:T**

   Deep vein thrombosis is an important postoperative complication, especially following pelvic and lower limb surgery. A number of risk factors have been described-age, obesity, varicose veins, immobility, pregnancy, Puerperium, high dose oestrogen therapy, previous DVT or pulmonary embolism, thrombophilia, deficiencies of anti-thrombin III, Protein C or S, trauma or surgery(especially pelvic, hip or lower limb), malignancy, congestive heart failure, infection, etc.

7. **A:T, B:T, C:T, D:T, E:T**

   DVT is seen in 30% of surgical patients. Sixty-five percent of patients with below knee deep vein thrombosis (DVT) are asymptomatic. Calf tenderness, swelling, fever and a raised temperature in the postoperative patient should increase the suspicion of DVT.

8. **A:T, B:T, C:F, D:T, E:F**

   A ruptured Baker's cyst mimics DVT in many ways. Doppler ultrasound is a useful first line investigation. Ascending venogram may also help in localising the clot.

   The incidence of DVT can be reduced by simple measures. The use of graduated compression stockings and pneumatic foot pumps should be encouraged in postoperative patients. Early postoperative mobilisation should be commenced and high-risk patients, identified.

Low molecular weight heparin is commonly used for prophylaxis of the DVT.

Pulmonary embolism is an important and potentially fatal complication of lower limb DVT.

9. **A:F, B:T, C:T, D:F, E:F**

Virchow's triad refers to the factors leading to the DVT. It consists of endothelial damage, hypercoagulability and sluggish blood flow. It is used only in relation to DVT. Supraclavicular lymph node enlargement following carcinoma (Virchow's node) of the stomach suggests a secondary spread.

10. **A:F, B:F, C:T, D:F, E:T**

Steroids are known to cause important side effects. Delayed wound healing, skin and musculoskeletal changes, sodium and water retention along with other metabolic abnormalities are associated with long-term steroid therapy.

Steroids are used in conditions affecting pituitary and adrenal glands. Commonly used steroids in surgical patients are Hydrocortisone, Prednisolone, Dexamethasone, etc.

11. **A:T, B:F, C:T, D:T, E:F**

Sickle cell disease is a haematological disorder commonly seen in people of African origin. The normal haemoglobin A is replaced by haemoglobin S (HBS). There is sickling of the red blood cells, leading to increased blood viscosity and obstruction of blood flow in the vessels. The susceptibility to infections, especially *Streptococcus pneumoniae* increases in the presence of splenic infarcts, due to sickle cell disease. Adequate oxygenation and hydration are essential throughout surgery. Blood transfusion may be necessary. In some patients, splenectomy is required.

The 'sickle cell crisis' is the thrombosis in the vessels caused by the sickling of the red blood cells due to abnormal haemoglobin.

12. **A:T, B:F, C:T, D:T, E:F**

Informed consent is an important part in the management of surgical patients. All surgeons must be familiar with the processes and details in the document before seeking agreement to proceed with any intervention. Consent involves a dialogue between surgeon and patient which leads to the signing of the consent form.

Medicolegally, the consent is invalid if signed by somebody other than the patient. But the parents of children below 16 years of age are allowed to sign a consent form on their behalf. A child of 13 years or above is also allowed to give an informed consent, if he or she is able to understand the risks and benefits of the procedure.

13. **A:F, B:F, C:T, D:F, E:T**

The pulse oximeter uses the technique of spectro-photometry and plethysmography to determine oxygen saturation of the arterial blood.

Pulse oximetry is a noninvasive procedure and actually measures only the saturation of the peripheral blood. Human oxyhaemoglobin and deoxyhaemoglobin have fixed patterns of absorbency for red and infrared light, so oxygen saturation of haemoglobin can be measured assuming constant haemoglobin concentration.

An oxygen saturation value of 95% or greater by pulse oximetry is strong corroborative evidence of adequate peripheral arterial oxygenation.

Partial pressure of oxygen in the blood can only be reliably measured by arterial blood gas analysis. Movement, poor application of the probe, peripheral vasoconstriction (low temperature), abnormal haemo-globin (carboxyhaemoglobin), jaundice and excessive ambient light may alter the measurements significantly.

The pulse oximeter probe is usually applied over the digits or earlobe.

14. **A:F, B:F, C:T, D:T, E:T**

    Malignant hyperthermia is a very rare condition of autosomal dominant inheritance. It is characterised by hyperthermia, muscle rigidity, tachycardia, tachypnoea and DIC. Metabolic acidosis, hyperkalaemia and renal failure may follow. It may respond to prompt treatment with Dantrolene sodium. Supportive measures like surface cooling and intravenous fluids are also required. Early identification is important as it is a potentially life-threatening condition. It is important to remember that any inhalational anaesthetic may induce 'malignant hyperthermia'.

15. **A:F, B:T, C:T, D:T, E:F**

    Premedication drugs prescribed by the anaesthetists are aimed to allay anxiety, dry secretions and provide analgesia. Benzodiazepines are known to cause anxiolysis and are commonly prescribed preoperatively.

    Opioid analgesics provide analgesia and also have excellent sedative properties.

    The drying of oral secretions is not usually necessary, nowadays. However, procedures like dental surgery, bronchoscopy or surgery in the lung for paediatric patients may require a drying agent such as Atropine or Hyoscine.

16. **A:F, B:T, C:F, D:F, E:F**

    'Relaxants' are used to provide relaxation of muscles during anaesthesia.

    There are 2 groups:'depolarising' and 'nondepolarising' muscle relaxants. Suxamethonium, is a commonly used depolarising muscle relaxant but it is associated with several side effects.

    Non-depolarising muscle relaxants are recommended because of few side effects, quick time of onset (2-3 minutes) and a reasonable duration of action (20 minutes to an hour). They competitively inhibit the acetylcholine receptors and muscle end plates, thus, blocking the acetylcholine action. Common non-depolarising agents are d-Tubocurarine, Alcuronium Pancuronium, Vecuronium and Atracurium.

The muscle relaxants, in general, do not have any intrinsic anaesthetic effect. Atracurium and Vecuronium are short-acting depolarising agents which are used as infusions for long cases and in intensive care.

17. **A:T, B:F, C:T, D:T, E:F**

Tourniquets are very commonly used in orthopaedic surgery. However, they should be used with caution as serious complications may occur following prolonged compression. The limb should be exsanguinated before the tourniquet is applied. Reperfusion period is about 90 and 120 minutes for upper and lower limbs, respectively. After this period, the tourniquet should be deflated to allow perfusion of the limb, thus avoiding the risk of ischaemia.

Tourniquets can precipitate a sickle cell crisis in individuals predisposed to this condition. This occurs mainly due to a reduction in the oxygen content of the blood distal to the tourniquet.

The pressure in the cuff of the tourniquet should never exceed 75 mmHg and 100 mmHg above the systolic pressure in the upper and lower limbs, respectively.

A ring tourniquet may be used for surgery on fingers. A good haemostasis is achieved with when the divided 'finger' of the latex gloves is rolled down to the base of the affected finger.

18. **A:T, B:F, C:F, D:T, E:T**

Suxamethonium is a depolarising relaxant used primarily for difficult intubation and crash induction. It is structurally similar to the acetylcholine molecule. Due to its short life (5-10 minutes) it is considered useful for very short surgical procedures in addition to crash induction and intubation. However, it is known to cause serious side effects like histamine-release, bradycardia, generalised somatic pain, hyperkalaemia, persistent neuromuscular blockade and malignant hyperthermia.

'Scoline apnoea' is caused by the prolonged action of suxamethonium due to an absent or abnormal plasma pseudocholinesterase. It is a genetically determined condition.

19. **A:T, B:T, C:F, D:T, E:F**
Local anaesthetics have membrane stabilising properties. They block the sodium channels in the axon membrane preventing inflow of sodium ions, which is necessary for propagation for impulses. The commonly used local anaesthetics are Lignocaine, Prilocaine, Bupivacaine and Cocaine.

The local anaesthetics, in general, are known to cause toxic effects on the CNS and CVS on systemic absorption. Few of these side effects like fits, coma, hypotension, and cardiac arrhythmias may be fatal.

The predominant effect of local anaesthetics is seen on C-fibres which conduct pain and are more sensitive than motor fibres in the A-group.

The maximum safe dose of Lignocaine is 3 mg/kg body weight and 5 mg/kg body weight when used with Adrenaline. The addition of Adrenaline prolongs the duration of action and slows systemic absorption. However, the combination of Adrenaline and Lignocaine is strongly contraindicated when infiltration is required close to end-arteries, for example, digits and penis as this may cause ischaemic necrosis.

20. **A:F, B:F, C:T, D:F, E:T**
The duration of action of Bupivacaine is longer than Lignocaine. It is commonly used for epidural and spinal anaesthesia. Its predominant toxic effects are seen in the cardiovascular system because it has a high affinity for cardiac muscle cells.

Bupivacaine is not recommended for intravenous use. The maximum safe dose is 3 mg/kg body weight with and 2 mg/kg body weight without Adrenaline. It may also be used for postoperative wound infiltration for prolonged analgesia.

21. **A:T, B:F, C:T, D:F, E:F**

Central venous pressure is a numerical value that represents the right atrial pressure (Normal 0-5 mmHg).

A value greater than 10 mmHg represents fluid overload or cardiac failure. The central venous pressure is recorded by the introduction of a catheter preferably through the internal jugular or subclavian veins (right more common than the left). The tip of the catheter should be placed in the superior vena cava for accurate measurement.

Central venous lines are indicated in critically ill patients and major surgery if problems are anticipated postoperatively. Besides measuring the pressure on the right side of the heart, the central venous catheter is also used for the administration of total parenteral nutrition and chemotherapy, haemodialysis and in some cases, where peripheral venous access is difficult. It is an invasive procedure and strict asepsis is recommended. Infection, pneumothorax, incorrect placement, nerve injury, thoracic duct injury, air embolism and other complications may occur following the introduction of the central venous catheter.

22. **A:T, B:T, C:F, D:T, E:T**

The pulmonary artery catheter also known as Swan-Ganz catheter (or pulmonary artery floatation catheter) is used to measure the catheter on the left side of the heart. It is a multi-luminal catheter with an inflatable balloon at the tip that ultimately wedges into the pulmonary artery after introduction. The cardiac output (thermal dilution), systemic vascular resistance, pulmonary vascular resistance and oxygen consumption on delivery, can easily be derived from the pulmonary artery catheter measurements. The normal value of pulmonary artery pressure is 6-12 mmHg. It is indicated in surgical patients having complex procedures and a complicated cardiac history, left ventricular failure, interstitial pulmonary oedema, valvular heart disease, critically ill patients and other situations where it is difficult to accurately judge the haemodynamic status. The catheter is introduced into a central vein and connected to an oscilloscope and advanced into the right atrium. Further, it is floated into the right ventricle and then into the pulmonary artery.

23. **A:F, B:T, C:F, D:F, E:T**
Diathermy is the passage of a high frequency alternating electric current AC through the body tissues. Very high local temperatures up to 1000°C, are generated.

Monopolar diathermy, which involves the use of a plate electrode, is more popular as it generates high power (400 watts) and unlike bipolar diathermy, can be used for cutting and cauterising bleeding vessels which are held by ordinary surgical forceps.

However, the bipolar diathermy (Power only about 50 watts) does not employ the use of patient electrode and the current passes between the 2 limbs of the diathermy forceps only. It is also inherently safer and is useful for surgery on the penis or digits.

The common cause of burns due to diathermy is incorrect application of the patient's plate, contact of the patient with metal objects and careless technique.

Safety measures should be employed to prevent burns to the patient and the operating surgeon has an overall responsibility for the safety of the diathermy.

24. **A:F, B:F, C:T, D:T, E:F**
Sterilisation is defined as the complete destruction of all viable organisms, including spores, viruses and mycobacteria. On the other hand, 'disinfection' is a process of reduction in the number of viable organisms but some viruses and bacterial spores may still remain active.

The various methods for sterilisation that are generally used are steam, hot air, ethylene oxide, low temperature steam and formaldehyde (LTSF) and irradiation.

Sterilisation by steam under pressure is one of the most commonly used procedures. Pressurised steam can kill bacteria, viruses and heat resistant spores.

Ethylene oxide is highly penetrative and ideal for heat sensitive equipment like rubber and plastic, sutures and single used items and other theatre equipment.

Gamma irradiation is an industrial process of sterilisation suitable for catheters, syringes, etc.

Sterilisation by low temperature steam and formaldehyde (LTSF) has the advantage of sterilisation at a low temperature (73°C) and is, therefore, useful for heat sensitive equipment and plastic items.

**25. A:F, B:F, C:T, D:F, E:F**

The history and clinical findings suggest the diagnosis of postoperative myocardial infarction in this patient. The points in favour are the nature and site of pain, presence of risk factors and tachycardia. Cardiac enzymes in the serum and the ECG can be normal in the initial stages and, therefore, they should be checked again after a few hours.

Although a diagnosis of pulmonary embolism cannot be completely ruled out, the clinical picture, arterial blood gases and other findings do not correspond with it. Hence, an urgent V/Q scan or anticoagulation is not necessary. This patient actually requires high flow oxygen, pain relief and close monitoring to establish a diagnosis and start definitive treatment. A medical opinion should be sought as soon as possible. Serum cardiac enzymes, arterial blood gases and an ECG should be repeated within the next few hours to assess the changes. It is important to note that postoperative MI commonly presents 3 days after surgery.

**26. A:F, B:T, C:T, D:F, E:F**

The time of onset of postoperative pyrexia may, sometimes, help in determining the cause. However, variations may be seen.

Pyrexia within 24 hours of any major surgery may be regarded as normal but still close monitoring is required because early intervention can alter the course of the underlying problem.

Pyrexia within 48 hours of surgery is highly suggestive of a chest infection especially in the presence of signs and symptoms in the chest.

Patients with deep vein thrombosis develop postoperative pyrexia at about the 10th day. Wound infection or anastomotic leak after a bowel resection and anastomosis causes a high temperature 5 to 7 days after surgery. Therefore, examination of wound is recommended in all cases presenting with a temperature, postoperatively.

27. **A:F, B:T, C:F, D:T, E:F**
The risk of DVT (and possible PE) is high in this patient due to age, HRT treatment, malignancy and obesity. Her clinical, radiological and arterial blood gas findings strongly suggest the diagnosis of pulmonary embolism. The improvement in the oxygen saturation on 100% oxygen further supports the diagnosis. This lady needs an urgent medical opinion and anticoagulation.

A ventilation perfusion scan would further support the diagnosis and, therefore, should be organised, as soon as possible. Close monitoring and frequent arterial blood gas sampling is necessary for further assessment. Radiotherapy and chemotherapy are not indicated in this situation.

28. **A:F, B:F, C:T, D:T, E:T**
Blood transfusion is associated with several complications: Congestive cardiac failure, transfusion reactions, transmission of infection like HIV, Hepatitis B, thrombophlebitis, embolism, coagulation failure (dilution of clotting factors and platelets, disseminated intravascular coagulation), hyperthermia, hyperkalaemia, citrate toxicity, acidosis, etc. Hyperkalaemia, is particularly seen after a massive blood transfusion due to the excess release of the potassium ions from the lysed RBC cells. There is a shift of the oxyhaemoglobin curve to the left due to a fall in the level of 2, 3-diphosphoglycerate in the stored cells. The affinity of

haemoglobin for oxygen increases, resulting in a shift of the oxyhaemoglobin curve to the left.

Platelets, factor VIII and factor V are deficient in stored blood, hence coagulation abnormalities may be seen after a massive transfusion of the stored blood.

Disseminated intravascular coagulation may occur following incompatible blood transfusion.

Transfusion reactions usually occur in the form of incompatibility or allergic reactions. They are immunologically mediated. Incompatibility mainly results from human error and may be avoided by careful grouping and cross matching.

29. **A:F, B:F, C:T, D:F, E:T**

Non-steroidal anti-inflammatory drugs (NSAIDs), especially Diclofenac, are commonly used on the medical and surgical wards for the treatment of pain. The main mechanism of action is by inhibition of prostaglandins, which are responsible for producing pain.

NSAIDs are known to cause serious side effects: Gastric ulceration, renal damage, bleeding, broncho-spasm, drug interactions (e.g. Warfarin) etc. Metabolic abnormalities (acidosis, metabolic acidosis and respiratory alkalosis) may also be seen. NSAIDs are administered either orally or per rectally. Opioid analgesics act on three main types of receptors—μ/κ/ Δ. Morphine and pethidine act on μ1 and μ2 receptors, respectively.

30. **A:F, B:T, C:F, D:T, E:F**

Postoperative hypoxaemia can adversely affect all the systems of the body. The intellectual functions may be impaired and progressive confusion is common, especially in the elderly patients.

Hypoxia has major cardiovascular effects. Hypoxaemia and tachycardia are known to be associated with myocardial ischaemia (myocardial infarction). As $PO_2$ falls below the level of 60 mmHg, there is a gradual rise in ventilation followed by an increase in oxygen consumption and a greater production of carbon dioxide.

Postoperative hypoxaemia is also known to cause poor wound healing in addition to haematological, GI, hepatic and renal dysfunctions.

31. **A:T, B:F, C:T, D:F, E:T**
Carbon monoxide is present as carboxyhaemoglobin (COHB) in the blood. The levels of COHB are very high in smokers. Carboxyhaemoglobin reduces the binding of haemoglobin to oxygen and also inhibits the ability of haemoglobin to give up oxygen to the tissues. Carbon monoxide has a negative ionotropic effect as well. Nicotine increases the heart rate and systemic arterial blood pressure. Stopping smoking even for 24 hours significantly reduces the level of COHB in blood.

32. **A:T, B:F, C:F, D:F, E:T**
Arterial blood gas is a useful tool for the assessment of the gases and ions in blood. It gives relatively accurate values of partial pressure of oxygen and its saturation in the arterial blood. Metabolic abnormalities like pH changes, acidosis and alkalosis, base deficits, etc can be determined by analysing an arterial blood gas sample. A high local temperature or a delay in the analysis of the withdrawn sample may affect the final results. The air in the syringe should be expelled after withdrawing the sample, which is inserted into the machine without delay, after mixing.

33. **A:F, B:T, C:T, D:F, E:F**
The calculation of oxygen delivery is very important in the management of the critically ill patients. Oxygen delivery is calculated as a product of cardiac output and oxygen content.
Oxygen delivery = CO × (constant × [Hb] × $SAO_2$) + dissolved oxygen or
Oxygen delivery = 5 litres per minute × (1.34ml/g × 150g/l × 0.97)
= 5 litres/min × approx 200ml/l
= 1,000ml/min at rest (600ml/min/m²).

It may be noted that cardiac output is a product of heart rate and/volume. Any change in heart rate/volume, haemoglobin or $SAO_2$ affects the oxygen delivery to the tissues. Stress in the form of exercise, trauma or surgery increases the oxygen demand and hence affects the oxygen delivery. The oxygen delivery as calculated above is about 1,000ml/min at rest.

34. **A:T, B:T, C:T, D:F, E:T**

Postoperatively, there may be a significant fall in the blood pressure. During the first postoperative day, haemorrhage is one of the most important causes. The haemorrhage may be primary or reactionary. In all cases the patient should be adequately resuscitated. Blood transfusion and re-exploration of the wound may be considered.

Drugs and septicaemia may cause postoperative hypotension by inducing vasodilatation. Myocardial infarction, which is another important cause of postoperative hypotension, reduces cardiac output leading to a fall in the arterial blood pressure.

Deep vein thrombosis in itself does not cause hypotension but the subsequent development of a pulmonary embolism may result in a haemodynamic collapse if the outflow to the right ventricle is obstructed.

35. **A:T, B:T, C:F, D:T, E:T**

Pulmonary embolism occurs following dislodgement of a venous thrombus generally from the lower limb veins. It is an important cause of sudden postoperative death. Common clinical features are pleuritic chest pain, shortness of breath, hypotension, haemoptysis, cyanosis, raised JVP, pleural rub and loud P2. Classically, it occurs 10 days after the operation. The patient has a rapid and thready pulse and may have a low blood pressure. The ECG may show sinus tachycardia and there may be a deep S wave in limb lead 1, Q and inverted T waves in limb lead 3 (the classical S1 Q3 T3 pattern). The chest X-ray is often normal and the blood gases may suggest a hypoxic picture. A ventilation perfusion (V/Q) scan of the lung will show areas of mismatch and pulmonary angiography may be considered. The treatment consists of adequate oxygenation, pain relief, Heparinisation and Warfarinisation. This complication can be prevented by early mobilisation, use of compression stockings, pneumatic pumps and low molecular weight (LMW) subcutaneous heparin, preoperatively.

36. **A:F, B:F, C:T, D:T, E:F**

Sutures in surgical practice are classified as absorbable or non-absorbable. The commonly used absorbable sutures are Vicryl (polyglactin), PDS (poly dioxanone), catgut and dexon.

Examples of non-absorbable sutures are polypropylene (prolene), polyamide, polyester, silk, stainless steel wire, etc.

Sutures are also classified as monofilament or multi-filament, braided or twisted, natural or synthetic.

An ideal suture should have a minimal inflammatory reaction, sufficient inside strength, good knotting and handling properties.

37. **A:T, B:T, C:F, D:T, E:T**

Bleeding disorders cause a disturbance in the clotting mechanism and, therefore, lead to bleeding tendencies. Measuring the FBC, APTT, PT, TT, fibrinogen, FDP levels and platelet count can help in screening these clotting disorders.

Administration of factors VIII and IX is indicated in congenital bleeding disorders.

The liver disorders cause a disruption in the production of the clotting factors and, therefore, the clotting mechanism is adversely affected. Both PT and APTT are increased while TT is usually, normal. Platelet count is decreased.

Warfarin, which is an anticoagulant, also increases PT, APTT but has no effect on TT and platelet counts.

Diazepam is not known to cause any abnormal bleeding tendencies.

In disseminated intravascular coagulation, the clotting cascade is activated and leads to an elevation in the PT, APTT, TT and a fall in the platelet count.

Factor VIII deficiency, also known as haemophilia, is a congenital X-linked recessive disorder and causes varying degrees of bleeding tendencies. Haemophilia B (deficiency of factor IX) and von Willebrand's disease (deficiency of von Willebrand factor vWF) are other common disorders that cause bleeding. Unlike haemophilia A and B, which are X-linked disorders, von Willebrand's disease is usually an autosomal dominant condition. However, autosomal recessive variants are also seen.

38. **A:F, B:F, C:F, D:T, E:F**
Keloid scars are formed by abnormal collagen metabolism and they seem to grow beyond the limits of the original wound. They may be familial, more common in blacks than whites and the common sites are sternum, shoulder and extensor surfaces. They often occur in wounds that have healed perfectly well without any complications. The best cure rates are achieved with a combination of surgery and postoperative interstitial radiotherapy. The application of pressure and intra-lesional injections of steroids such as Triamcinolone can also prove helpful.

On the other hand, the hypertrophic scars are more common on the flexor surfaces, have spontaneous resolution and are confined to the limits of the original wound.

39. **A:T, B:F, C:F, D:F, E:T**
The pH of the blood is the negative logarithm of the hydrogen ion concentration. The normal value ranges from 7.36 to 7.44. Acidosis denotes a fall in the pH from the normal range while alkalosis indicates a pH higher than 7.44. The pH of the blood is regulated by various

buffering mechanisms, for example bicarbonate to carbonic acid ratio. This ratio remains fairly constant through the compensatory mechanisms.

40. **A:T, B:T, C:F, D:F, E:T**

| | |
|---|---|
| pH | 7.36-7.44 (44-36nmol l⁻¹) |
| $PCO_2$ | 4.6-5.6 kPa (35-42 mmHg) |
| $PO_2$ | 10-13 kPa (75-100 mmHg) |
| $HCO_3$ | 22-26 mmol l⁻¹ |
| SBC | 22-26 mol l⁻¹ |
| Base excess | -2 to + 2 nmol l⁻¹ |
| Standard base excess | -3 to + 3 nmol l⁻¹ |
| $O_2$ saturation | > 95% |

41. **A:F, B:T, C:F, D:T, E:T**

The normal daily requirement of water in a 70kg adult is about 35ml/kg body weight (total 2,500 ml). The daily requirement of each of the principle ions of the body, namely, sodium, potassium and chloride is 1 mmol/kg body weight (70 mmol). The requirement of calcium and magnesium is nearly equal (0.1 mmol/kg body weight-total 7 mmol).

0.2 mmol/kg body weight (14 mmol) is the approximate requirement for phosphate iron in the body.
[These figures are easy to remember:
$(1 \rightarrow 2 \rightarrow 7 \rightarrow 14 \rightarrow 35 \rightarrow 70)$].

42. **A:F, B:T, C:F, D:F, E:T**

All patients undergoing surgery develop a metabolic response to the injury that is proportional to the severity of the surgical insult. A part of this response is basically an adaptive response to maintain homeostasis in the body. There is a reduction in the glomerular filtration rate following surgery. Tubular resorption of sodium is enhanced following an increase in the aldosterone secretion. Water is retained due to enhanced production of ADH and also inability to excrete free water or hypotonic urine. Pain and blood loss causes vasoconstriction in the renal vessels.

Protein catabolism is an important metabolic response to surgery and leads to the formation of nitrogenous waste products.

43. **A:F, B:T, C:F, D:T, E:F**
The total body water is 45 litres. One-third of this is in the extracellular compartment whilst the other two-thirds is present as intracellular fluid. Of the 15 litres present in the extracellular compartment (one-third of total body water), plasma constitutes 3.5 litres, interstitial fluid (tissue fluid) 8.5 litres, lymph 1.5 litres and transcellular fluid 1.5 litres. Two-thirds of the total body water is present as intracellular fluid, which is about 30 litres. Sixty percent of the total body weight equals total body water.

CSF, intraocular, pleural, digestive secretions, synovial and gut fluid form the transcellular fluid.
Interstitial fluid = Extracellular fluid − intravascular volume.

44. **A:T, B:T, C:F, D:F, E:F**
Hartmann's solution, also known as Ringer's lactate contains 131, 111, 5 mmol/litre of sodium, chloride and potassium ions, respectively. This solution along with normal saline and 5% dextrose are the common intravenous fluids prescribed in the perioperative period. The sodium content of Ringer's lactate is lower than that of normal saline (131 against 150). In prescribing any fluid regimen the basal requirements, continuing abnormal losses over and above basal requirements and pre-existing dehydration and electrolyte loss should be calculated to provide adequate fluid replacement.

45. **A:T, B:T, C:T, D:T, E:F**
Several surgical and medical causes may precipitate hypokalaemia, e.g. inadequate intake, gastrointestinal losses (vomiting, diarrhoea, fistula losses), diuretics (especially thiazide group), Cushing syndrome, etc.

Muscle weakness, hypotonia, cardiac arrhythmias, cramps and tetany may be seen following hypokalaemia.

Potassium levels less than 2.5 mmol/l are dangerous and should be urgently treated. Mild derangement can be corrected by oral supplementation of potassium while intravenous administration is necessary in more severe cases. However, potassium should never be given as a rapid bolus IV injection as it may cause asystole and cardiac arrest.

The normal value for serum potassium is 3.5 to 5.5 mmol/l.

46. **A:F, B:F, C:T, D:T, E:F**

Vitamin K is a fat-soluble vitamin and its absorption may be impaired in the hepatobiliary disease. Vitamin K is responsible for the hepatic synthesis of coagulation factors II, VII, IX and X. Deficiency of vitamin K may lead to serious bleeding tendencies. PT and APTT are increased while TT and platelet counts may be normal.

Parenteral administration of vitamin K should be considered in patients with biliary obstruction.

47. **A:F, B:F, C:F, D:T, E:F**

Inflammation causes a rise in the production of prostaglandins. The cell membrane phospholipids are converted into arachidonic acid by the action of phospholipase. Arachidonic acid metabolism through the cyclo-oxygenase pathway produces prostaglandins and thromboxane A2.

Important prostaglandins are $PGI_2$, $PGE_2$, $PG_2$. In general they cause vasodilatation, platelet aggregation, high temperature and leucocytosis.

Aspirin inhibits the production of prostaglandins by directly affecting the cyclo-oxygenase enzyme.

Leukotrines are the breakdown products of arachidonic acid through the 'lipoxygenase pathway'. They cause chemotaxis, vasoconstriction, broncho-constriction and increased vascular permeability.

The nucleated cells, except lymphocytes, mainly produce prostaglandins.

48. **A:T, B:T, C:T, D:F, E:F**

Tumour necrosis factor alpha (also known as cachectin) is released from the macrophages by the action of the bacterial endotoxin. It is a potent cytokine known to cause anorexia, tachypnoea, fever and tachycardia. It has profound effects on fibroblast proliferation and neutrophil activation. It also stimulates the production of other cytokines, ACTH, APR and affects the body metabolism in many ways.

High concentrations of TNF-α may cause multiple organ dysfunction syndrome. It also possesses antiviral effects.

49. **A:T, B:T, C:F, D:T, E:T**

Interferons are of various types:alpha, beta and gamma. Leucocytes and fibroblasts produce alfa and beta interferons, respectively; while the gamma interferon is produced by antigen-activated lymphocytes. In general, they synergise with other cytokines, inhibit viral replication, enhance MHC expression and improve cytotoxicity against certain target cancer cells. Gamma interferon is said to inhibit prostaglandin release.

50. **A:F, B:T, C:F, D:F, E:T**

Interleukin-6 is an important inflammatory cytokine. It is produced by the macrophages, fibroblasts, mast cells and T-cells. It has a prominent action on the immune and haemopoietic systems. It is also a B-cell growth factor and is, therefore, involved in the production of plasma cells. The growth of the malignant myeloma cells is enhanced due to the stimulation provided by the cytokine Interleukin-6.

51. **A:F, B:F, C:T, D:T, E:F**

Hypersensitivity reactions involve the activation of immune response to an exogenous antigen. Various types of hypersensitivity reactions are described:Type I to Type V.

Common examples are:

Type I - hay fever

Type II - drug reactions

Type III - acute glomerulonephritis

Type IV - immune response in tuberculosis and transplant rejection

Type V - myasthenia gravis.

Type IV hypersensitivity reaction is mediated by the sensitised T-lymphocytes and is also known as delayed hypersensitivity reaction. The release of cytokines from the T-helper cells causes the activation of macrophage and monocytes leading to extensive cell damage.

52. **A:F, B:F, C:T, D:T, E:F**

Wound healing can be divided into 3 stages: inflammation, cell proliferation and matrix formation (matrix remodelling).

It may also be classified according to the mechanism with approximation of the wound edges, i.e. primary, secondary and tertiary intentions. A wound is said to heal by primary intention when the edges are in close apposition that may have been achieved by the use of sutures or staples.

The wounds that heal with secondary intention have extensive loss of epithelium and a large sub-epithelial tissue defect may also be present. Such wounds may heal with bad looking scars.

Healing by tertiary intention (delayed primary closure) is achieved when the granulation tissue has formed and a proper closure of the wound is instituted.

Cytokines, Interleukin-1 and tumour necrosis factor alpha have significant roles in wound healing. IL-1 causes dermal fibroblast proliferation and appropriate regulation of collagen synthesis by the fibroblast. The tumour necrosis factor alpha is the main factor responsible for causing wasting and tumour cell death. It also promotes ingrowth of new blood vessels in the healing wounds. The growth factors including platelet derived growth actor (PDGF), epidermal growth factor (EGF) and transforming growth factor alpha and beta (TGF-α and β) also have significant roles in wound healing. Malnutrition, administration of steroids, presence of infection, ischaemic and hypoxia can all adversely affect wound healing.

53. **A:T, B:T, C:T, D:F, E:T**
Surgical wounds may be classified as clean (class I), clean contaminated (class II), contaminated (class III) and dirty (class IV) on the basis of the rate of infection in the wound. The rate of infection in a clean wound should not exceed 2%; clean contaminated about 5%; contaminated about 20%. The wounds are classified as dirty or class IV if the rate of infection is up to 40%.

The wound dehiscence is a disruption in any layer of the operative wound. An underlying infection may be the cause.

Wound contraction is a process by which the wound shortens during healing. This is brought about by myofibroblasts that are actually cells possessing features of fibroblasts and smooth muscle cells.

A badly infected wound should never be closed as the infection can track down the deeper layers. A secondary closure is carried out following the formation of a healthy granulation tissue.

Epithelialisation, contraction and connective tissue formation are the normal stages in the healing of any wound.

54. **A:T, B:F, C:T, D:T, E:T**
Wound dehiscence is the partial or total disruption in the layers of the operative wound. An impending wound dehiscence may present as a pink coloured discharge from the wound in the immediate postoperative period. In a high proportion of cases, wound infection may be the underlying problem. Other factors predisposing to wound infection are old age, respiratory diseases, obesity, malnutrition, steroid therapy, diabetes mellitus and malignancy.

Ischaemia and increased mobility at the site of the wound may also cause wound dehiscence. In some cases it may prove fatal, especially in those with haemodynamic compromise. Immediate resuscitative measures should be instituted with protection of organs with moist bags. Closure of the wound with stronger sutures should be considered as early as possible.

55. **A:T, B:F, C:T, D:T, E:F**
Total parenteral nutrition must be avoided where enteral feeding is possible and the GI tract is functioning normally.

TPN is associated with many important and serious compilations, e.g. displacement of catheter, infections, metabolic derangement, etc.

Total parenteral nutrition is only used in a small percentage of patients (about 4-5% of all hospital admissions). It is only used in cases where enteric feeding is not possible or as a supplementation to enteral feeding in some cases. It may cause deficiency or excess of blood glucose, sodium, potassium, and calcium. Deficiency of vitamins and trace elements is also seen.

Regular monitoring of patients on nutritional support is essential for early identification of complications.

All patients should have daily full blood count, urea and electrolytes and random blood glucose; weekly liver function tests and levels of trace elements; assessment of vitamin $B_{12}$, zinc, magnesium, selenium and copper every 10-14 days.

56. **A:T, B:F, C:T, D:T, E:T**
Ventilation, critical illness, hypothyroidism, head injury, abdominal injury and diabetic neuropathy are known to cause gastric paresis (atony) by various mechanisms. Such patients should be considered for naso-duodenal or naso-jejunal feeding in order to minimise the risk of regurgitation or aspiration. If enteral feeding is not possible, the parenteral route should be considered. However, ideally, the decision to institute parenteral

nutrition should be taken in consultation with a multidisciplinary support team.

57. **A:T, B:F, C:T, D:T, E:F**
The nutritional status of a patient can be determined by a thorough history and clinical examination. Recent weight loss of more than 10%, serum albumin less than 30g/l, gross muscle wasting, peripheral oedema, major trauma, critical illness, etc are important indications for nutritional support. Both types of nutritional support—enteral and parenteral—may cause complications. However, the adverse effects following the administration of total parenteral nutrition are probably much more serious and difficult to manage. Patients on nutritional support with the enteral route can develop pulmonary aspiration, diarrhoea, vomiting, nausea, cramps, etc.

Complications following TPN may be immediate (e.g. those related to the insertion of the catheter, metabolic problems, etc) or late (e.g. infection, catheter displacement, etc) Therefore, parenteral nutrition requires very close monitoring and urgent action when complications develop.

58. **A:T, B:T, C:T, D:F, E:F**
Abdominal wound dehiscence is a serious complication and carries a high mortality rate. The patient should be adequately resuscitated before being taken to theatre. Re-exploration and peritoneal lavage may be necessary. Re-suturing of the wound should be done without any tension using non-absorbable monofilament sutures, for example PDS (polydioxanone) and a 'mass closure' is recommended.

59. **A:T, B:T, C:F, D:F, E:F**
Sepsis is defined as the systemic inflammatory response syndrome resulting from a proven infection. The temperature of the body may be high or low. There may be leukocytosis or leukopenia. In the initial stages, the urine output may be normal but later on, oliguria or anuria develops, depending upon the severity of the

condition. The mental faculties may be affected. Confusion, drowsiness, depressed levels of conscious-ness are prominent features in the well established cases.

Blood cultures are sterile in approximately 50% of patients with sepsis as the reaction is actually mediated by the cytokines and not by the pathogen, itself.

Proper oxygenation of the patient is necessary and ventilation may be required. Adequate fluid resuscitation with crystalloids, colloids and blood as indicated should be instituted. Inotropic support may be required to combat the shock. Antibiotic therapy and surgical drainage may become necessary depending on the cause of the condition.

60. **A:T, B:T, C:F, D:T, E:F**

61. **A:T, B:T, C:F, D:T, E:F**
Helicobacter pylori is a spiral shaped gram-negative organism and has known associations with duodenal ulcers, gastric ulcers, type B antral gastritis and possibly B cell MALT lymphoma and gastric cancer. It can be diagnosed by urea breath test, histopathological examination, serology, mucosal biopsy and culture. It causes mucosal damage and enhances the formation of hydrochloric acid by different mechanisms leading to ulceration of the intestinal mucosa. Triple therapy is recommended for its eradication. This consists of a week's course of a proton pump inhibitor plus Amoxycillin/Clarithromycin and Metronidazole.

Helicobacter pylori, characteristically causes the hydrolysis of urea resulting in the production of ammonia which is a strong alkali. This stimulates the secretion of gastrin from the antral G cells resulting in hypergastrinaemia and subsequent hyper secretion of the acid.

CLO test is a commercial urea test and utilises the ability of this organism to hydrolyse the urea. It is useful in the identification of the organism.

The recurrence of *H. pylori* infection is quite low after eradication with the triple regimen.

62. **A:T, B:F, C:F, D:F, E:T**
Gram-negative organisms like *E. coli* are the major causative organisms in septic shock and certain gastro-intestinal infections. The Clostridium group of organisms cause tetanus and gas gangrene; cellulitis is due to Streptococcal infections.

63. **A:2, B:1, C:3, D:4, E:8**
*Haemophilus influenzae* is the commonest organism causing osteomyelitis in children less than 4 years of age.
   30-40% cases of subacute bacterial endocarditis are caused by *Streptococcus viridans*.
   High temperature, malaise headache, diarrhoea, splenomegaly, etc are common features in infections with salmonella organisms. Perforation of an intestinal ulcer is an important complication of salmonella infection. Ileus may also occur.
   *Clostridium tetani* causes muscle spasm and rigidity due to the release of 'tetanospasmin' which is an exotoxin.
   Hidradenitis suppurativa commonly occurs in females in the second or third decades of life. Ducts of the apocrine glands are blocked, subsequently leading to infection, commonly by Bacteroides.
   Exotoxin is a protein with strong antigenic properties. It is heat labile, highly specific in its action and usually, produced by the gram-positive bacteria (e.g. 'tetanospasmin'from *Clostridium tetani*).

64. **A:F, B:F, C:T, D:T, E:T**
*Clostridium tetani* is a typical example of exotoxin.
   Gram-positive bacteria usually produce the exotoxins. They are highly antigenic, composed of protein and heat labile in nature. They have very specific actions and are neutralised by the antibodies.

65. **A:T, B:F, C:F, D:F, E:F**
Cefuroxime is a second generation cephalosporins with a wide range of activity against gram-positive and negative bacteria. It is very useful in surgical prophylaxis (e.g. joint replacement surgery).

Less than 10% of penicillin patients are also hyper-sensitive to Cephalosporins. Hypersensitivity, gastro-intestinal disturbances, hepato and nephro-toxicity, haematological disturbances, etc are the common complications of cefuroxime.

66. **A:F, B:T, C:F, D:T, E:F**
Leg amputations and wounds of warfare are at an increased risk of developing 'gas gangrene'. This condition is characterised by the growth of a group of anaerobic gas producing organisms in a badly damaged muscle. *Clostridium perfringens (welchii)* is involved in about 80% cases but other Clostridia may also be present. The alpha-toxin is considered important in the pathogenesis of gas gangrene. The traumatised muscle is involved in its entire length and develops a foul smelling necrosis leading to a dull appearance. Crepitus can be detected underneath muscle or the skin. The infection can spread through the blood into other organs, mainly the liver. The treatment consists of adequate resuscitation, antibiotics, and extensive debridement to remove the dead tissue. Hyperbaric oxygen may also be considered, when available. Characteristically, the wound is under tension and the overlying skin becomes discoloured.

67. **A:F, B:T, C:T, D:F, E:T**
Methicillin-resistant *Staphylococcus aureus* (MRSA) infections are difficult to manage. The common antibiotics fail to affect the bacterial cell wall synthesis of the multiplying organisms. Proper screening of the patient and staff with strict measures such as barrier nursing should be encouraged. Cross infection with MRSA can occur easily and may be seen in the ITU patients as well. Antibiotics like, Teicoplanin and Vancomycin, are commonly used to control MRSA infections but the treatment is very expensive.

68. **A:T, B:T, C:T, D:T, E:F**
    Systemic inflammatory response syndrome is a widespread inflammatory process consisting of two of the following features: hyperthermia more than 38°C, hypothermia less than 36°C, tachycardia more than 90 per minute, white cell count more than $12 \times 10^9$ /litre or less than $4 \times 10^9$ /litre. Systemic inflammatory response syndrome combined with proven infection constitutes 'sepsis' and 'severe sepsis or sepsis syndrome' is defined as sepsis in addition to one or more organ failure (for example, respiratory, cardiovascular, renal, etc).

69. **A:F, B:T, C:T, D:F, E:T**
    Strict asepsis must be ensured in all patients undergoing any type of total joint replacement surgery. Laminar airflow, three doses of prophylactic antibiotics and the absence of any focus of infection are standard requirements for joint replacement surgery. Urethral catheterization should be avoided as far as possible, as it may introduce infection. However, it can be used in some cases (e.g. epidural anaesthesia, monitoring of postoperative urinary output, etc)

70. **A:T, B:T, C:F, D:T, E:T**
    Surgeons operating on HIV patients are at an increased risk of acquiring the infection. However, risks can be minimised by observing certain general precautions. Double gloving provides a certain degree of protection against skin contamination from glove perforation.

    All sharp instruments and scalpels should be passed between the operative surgeon and the nurse in a kidney dish to reduce the risk of injury. There should be a minimum number of surgical assistants and the operation should be temporarily stopped if the position of the assistant needs to be changed.

    Preoperative identification of high-risk patients such as homosexuals, IV drug abusers, helps to alert the surgeon in advance. Adequate haemostasis should be achieved and alarming situations like unexpected bleeding should be avoided as they increase the risk of injury from surgeon to surgeon or surgeon to nurse following a quick response.

71. **A:F, B:T, C:T, D:F, E:T**

Necrotising fasciitis may be mono-microbial (group A beta-haemolytic Streptococci) or poly-microbial (anaerobes, coliforms, non group-A streptococci, etc). It is an infection that spreads along the facial planes involving the skin, subcutaneous tissue and deep fascia mainly. Common sites are the genitalia, groin and lower abdomen.

Necrotizing fasciitis may be associated with conditions like diabetes mellitus, malnutrition, obesity and immunocompromised states.

Clinically, the patient may show sudden deterioration. Areas of subcutaneous induration and erythema may develop. Treatment consists of resuscitation followed by extensive surgical debridement of the dead tissue. Antibiotics and supportive therapy must be instituted.

72. **A:2, B:5, C:7, D:6, E:1**

This young man has signs of cellulitis following an inset bite. It is usually caused by *Streptococcus pyogenes* and treatment with broad-spectrum antibiotics, initially intravenously and then orally, is generally successful.

'Carbuncle' is the subcutaneous infective gangrene caused by *Staphylococcus aureus*. It is commonly seen in diabetics. Antibiotics and surgical debridement are used to control the infection.

Kaposi's sarcoma is a malignant condition of the anal canal secondary to HIV infection. The hepatitis B vaccine provides satisfactory immunity against hepatitis B virus following initial three doses and then, a booster at 5 years.

*Clostridium defficile* infection is seen in the colonic mucosa after prolonged treatment with antibiotics.

There is formation of a pseudomembrane (hence, the name 'pseudomembranous colitis'). The changes can be detected by sigmoidoscopy and are mainly caused due to the release of a toxin by the C. *difficile* bacteria.

The bacteria may be cultured by the ELISA technique and the treatment involves cessation of the antibiotic therapy and commencement of oral Metronidazole or Vancomycin, if possible.

# 2

## Trauma and Critical Surgical Illness

1. A 42-year-old patient is found unconscious after a road traffic accident. His car is badly damaged and he has an actively bleeding wound in his right thigh, which looks deformed. The top priority in the management includes:
   A. Control of bleeding in the thigh
   B. Antibiotics
   C. Referral to neurosurgeons for a possible head injury
   D. Maintenance of airway and cervical spine immobilization
   E. Referral to orthopaedic surgeons and fracture stabilization

2. Intracranial pressure:
   A. Usually decreases in intracranial haemorrhage
   B. Normal value is 45 mmHg
   C. Can directly cause an increase in the cerebral perfusion when raised
   D. If normal in a trauma situation, excludes an intracranial haemorrhage
   E. If very high can cause herniation of brain

3. The Glasgow Coma Score of a patient with the following findings:
   • Abnormal flexion response to pain
   • Eye opening to the verbal commands
   • Inappropriate words
   A. 2
   B. 14
   C. 9
   D. 11
   E. 3

---

1. A:F, B:F, C:F, D:T, E:F     2. A:F, B:F, C:F, D:F, E:T
3. A:F, B:F, C:T, D:F, E:F

4. A young man is brought in to the accident and emergency department with multiple injuries after a road traffic accident. His pulse rate is 128 per minute and he has lost about 35% of his blood volume.
   A. Is in class III shock
   B. Needs resuscitation by crystalloids only
   C. Has lost more than 1500 ml of blood
   D. May also have a diminished urine output
   E. Blood pressure and pulse pressure should be markedly increased

5. The classic features of neurogenic shock include:
   A. Hypervolemia
   B. Cutaneous vasoconstriction without tachycardia
   C. Cutaneous vasoconstriction with tachycardia
   D. Narrowed pulse pressure
   E. Increased sympathetic tone

6. Hypovolemic shock:
   A. Results from a loss in the circulating volume, after haemorrhage, or loss of electrolytes, etc
   B. Causes bradycardia and vasodilatation, initially
   C. If class I, may be corrected by crystalloids alone
   D. Results in a rise in the cardiac output
   E. Never responds to a fluid challenge

7. Approximate blood loss:
   A. # Humerus     Max 50 ml
   B. # Pelvis      Upto 1000 ml
   C. # Femur       1000-2000 ml
   D. # Tibia       Upto 500 ml
   E. Open #        Amount may be doubled

---

4. A:T, B:F, C:T, D:T, E:F      5.  A:F, B:F, C:F, D:F, E:F
6. A:T, B:F, C:T, D:F, E:F      7.  A:F, B:F, C:T, D:T, E:T

8. **In haemorrhagic shock:**
    A. 0.1 ml/kg/hr is regarded as an adequate urine output for an adult
    B. 1 ml/kg/hr is an adequate urine output for the paediatric patient
    C. The peripheries are warm and the patient is bradycardic
    D. Adequate ventilatory exchange and oxygenation is the top priority
    E. Use of tourniquet is recommended for the control of bleeding

9. **Tension pneumothorax:**
    A. Must be confirmed radiologically before the treatment is instituted
    B. Definitive treatment involves the insertion of a chest drain
    C. May be easily confused with cardiac tamponade
    D. Is characterised by hypotension, hyperresonant chest and tracheal deviation
    E. Demands an urgent action

10. **Features of cardiac tamponade:**
    A. Beck's triad
    B. Kussmaul's sign
    C. Exaggerated pulsus paradoxus
    D. Muffled heart sounds
    E. Common after a blunt injury to the chest

11. **Chest drain:**
    A. Normally inserted in the 2nd or 3rd intercostals space anterior to the midaxillary line
    B. Needs to be checked with a chest X-ray after insertion
    C. Should be inserted through an incision just below the rib
    D. Radiologically evident haemothorax is an important indication
    E. Can lead to the development of thoracic empyema

8. A:F, B:T, C:F, D:T, E:F      9. A:F, B:T, C:T, D:T, E:T
10. A:T, B:T, C:T, D:T, E:F     11. A:F, B:T, C:F, D:T, E:T

12. **Rectal examination, in a trauma patient, is important to:**
    A. Assess sphincter tone
    B. Rule out BPH
    C. Confirm the presence of blood from GI perforation
    D. Assess a urethral injury
    E. Detect the presence of lumbar fractures

13. **Signs of intra-abdominal injury:**
    A. Involuntary guarding
    B. Rebound tenderness
    C. Diffuse dullness
    D. Bruit
    E. Enlarged liver

14. **Indications for laparotomy in a trauma patient:**
    A. Profound hypovolemia despite resuscitation
    B. Soft but slightly tender abdomen
    C. A major associated chest injury
    D. Stable pelvic fracture
    E. Free gas within the abdomen

15. **Head Injury:**
    A. CPP = Mean arterial pressure + Intracranial pressure
    B. GCS of 10 is classified as severe head injury
    C. Hyperventilation helps in the reduction of intracranial pressure
    D. IV fluid administration should be avoided
    E. Convex lenticular shadow on CT suggests subdural haematoma

16. **Basal skull fractures:**
    A. Otorrhoea is never seen
    B. Battle's sign denotes periorbital cellulitis
    C. Olfactory nerve palsy may occur frequently
    D. Bacterial meningitis may be a complication
    E. Should be confirmed with an X-ray

---

12. A:T, B:F, C:T, D:T, E:F        13. A:T, B:T, C:T, D:F, E:F
14. A:T, B:F, C:F, D:F, E:T        15. A:F, B:F, C:T, D:F, E:F
16. A:F, B:F, C:F, D:T, E:F

17. **Brown-Séquard syndrome:**
    A. Common complication in trauma patients
    B. Is associated with contralateral motor loss
    C. Is characterised by ipsilateral loss of sensations
    D. Involves hemisection of the cord
    E. Spinothalamic tract and the corticospinal tract, both are involved

18. **Crush syndrome:**
    A. Causes early hepatic failure
    B. Renal function is not affected
    C. May lead to hypercalcaemia
    D. IV fluids and osmotic diuresis are useful
    E. Results from a significant injury to the muscle

19. **Compartment syndrome:**
    A. May lead to Volkmann's ischaemic contracture
    B. May be ruled out if a good peripheral pulse is present
    C. Diagnosis is confirmed by an angiogram
    D. May occur following an application of a tight bandage or a plaster
    E. Is characterised by severe pain n the leg after passive dorsiflexon of the toes

20. **C-spine radiography in a suspected case of cervical injury:**
    A. Must include the base of skull, all cervical vertebrae and the first thoracic vertebra
    B. A lateral view is sufficient to rule out more than 95% of the injuries
    C. Is unsatisfactory in 95% cases and hence a CT scan is required in almost all the cases
    D. Is not necessary in a patient with only neck pain and no neurological features
    E. Should be never done in an unconscious patient

---

17. A:F, B:F, C:F, D:T, E:T      18. A:F, B:T, C:F, D:T, E:T
19. A:T, B:F, C:F, D:T, E:T      20. A:T, B:F, C:F, D:F, E:F

21. **Chance fracture:**
    A. Is an injury of the cervical spine
    B. May be associated with retroperitoneal and abdominal visceral injuries
    C. Occurs following distraction in flexion
    D. Is usually common in drivers not wearing a seat belt
    E. Is the same as a burst fracture

22. **Paediatric fluid resuscitation after trauma:**
    A. An initial bolus of 20ml/kg is usually recommended
    B. A urinary output of >0.1ml/kg/hr is considered a good response to the fluid resuscitation
    C. Intraosseous infusion may be considered if venous access fails in a 4-year-old child
    D. 3:1 rule does not apply to children
    E. Is based on the body weight

23. **Features of non-accidental injury in a child:**
    A. Single fracture after a fall
    B. Discrepancy between the history and physical findings
    C. A prolonged interval between injury and presentation to the doctor
    D. Multiple injuries of different age
    E. Burns in unusual areas

24. **A man develops a laceration in his forearm after being attacked with a knife. He is unable to grip a piece of paper between his fingers. He also develops a deformity at the fingers. The surgeon tells him that he has injured a nerve that helps in the extension of the IP joints of the digits while all the other nerves are intact. He, therefore, may also have:**
    A. Absent sensations in the dorsal aspect of first space
    B. Absent sensations in the index finger
    C. Positive Froment's sign
    D. Pointing index sign
    E. Absent sensation in the medial one and a half fingers

---

21. A:F, B:T, C:T, D:F, E:F
23. A:F, B:T, C:T, D:T, E:T

22. A:T, B:F C:T, D:F, E:T
24. A:F, B:F, C:T, D:F, E:T

25. **The ulnar nerve:**
    A. Is commonly injured in the fractures of the scaphoid
    B. Supplies the oblique head of the adductor pollicis through its superficial branch
    C. Is related to Gyon's canal
    D. Compression causes carpal tunnel syndrome
    E. Root value is $C_{7,8} T_1$

26. **Anterior cruciate ligament:**
    A. Injuries may give rise to a positive Lachman test
    B. Rupture commonly causes haemarthrosis few days after the injury
    C. Is attached to the tibial tubercle
    D. Is extra-articular
    E. Ruptures are associated with instability

27. **Salter Harris injuries:**
    A. Commonly occur in adults
    B. Type II is the most common type
    C. Are classified according to the position of the metaphyseal fragment
    D. Type I has a good prognosis
    E. Do not cause growth disturbance

28. **Sepsis:**
    A. Is characterised by a marked reduction in the level of cytokines
    B. Never causes alkalosis
    C. May activate coagulation pathway
    D. Causes a depression in the myocardial activity
    E. Mortality rate is more than 10%

---

25. A:F, B:F, C:T, D:F, E:T          26. A:T, B:F, C:F, D:F, E:T
27. A:F, B:T, C:F, D:T, E:F          28. A:F, B:F, C:T, D:T, E:T

29. **Thoracic trauma:**
    A. 25 year-old-with a sharp instrument inserted in the right side of the chest and rapid accumulation of 2 l of blood in the chest drain
    B. A young man with an open chest wound (6×5 cm) which when closed by an occlusive dressing on three sides causes improvement in the chest symptoms
    C. A 53-year-old lady involved in a road traffic accident with multiple rib fractures, hypoxia and paradoxical respiration
    D. A 48-year-old lady intubated and ventilated after a head injury develops a sudden collapse of the lung and hypotension after PPV
    E. An 18-year-old man with a penetrating injury on the left side of the chest with air hunger, distended veins, hypotension but no hyperresonance.

    1. Simple pneumothorax
    2. Massive haemothorax
    3. Tension pneumothorax
    4. Diaphragmatic injury
    5. Open pneumothorax
    6. Cardiac tamponade
    7. Flail chest

30. **Indications for ITU transfer of a surgical patient:**
    A. Respiratory failure requiring ventilation
    B. Advanced cardiovascular monitoring, e.g. pulmonary artery floatation cather and ionotropic support
    C. Urea = 13 mmol/l and creatinine 95 μmol/l on the first postoperative day
    D. A need for one to one nursing
    E. Osteomyelitis secondary to diabetic ulceration

---

29. A:2, B:5: C:7, D:3, E:6     30.   A:T, B:T, C:F, D:T, E:F

31. Complications of ventilation:
    A. Increase in venous return
    B. Barotrauma
    C. Respiratory alkalosis
    D. Water depletion due to ↓ secretion of vasopression
    E. Disuse atrophy of respiratory muscles

32. Blood results analysis in a postoperative patient (on 60% Oxygen) with a low urinary output
    pH =7.1, $PCO_2$= 3.7, $PaO_2$= 11.2, Std Bicarbonate =14.3, Base Excess = –13, Oxygen saturation = 89%, Hb= 9.8, WCC = 18.4, Neutrophils = 13.6 Plat 200 × 10$^{11}$:
    A. Primary derangement is metabolic alkalosis
    B. The patient is hypoventilating
    C. ITU admission not indicated
    D. Sepsis is unlikely
    E. Compensatory respiratory acidosis

33. In acute renal failure:
    A. Most common cause in postoperative patients is post-renal
    B. CVP lines and pulmonary artery floatation catheter may become necessary for monitoring
    C. Determination of hourly urinary output is unnecessary
    D. Hyperkalaemia is an important and potentially life-threatening biochemical abnormality
    E. Correction of dehydration is of primary importance in postoperative patients

34. In DIC:
    A. Sepsis is an important causative factor
    B. PT and PTT are markedly reduced
    C. Fibrinogen levels are typically low
    D. Thrombocytopenia is a common feature
    E. Thrombin activation is the key event

---

31. A:F, B:T, C:T, D:F, E:T      32. A:F, B:F, C:F, D:F, E:F
33. A:F, B:T, C:F, D:T, E:T      34. A:T, B:F, C:T, D:T, E:T

35. **Oxygen dissociation curve:**
    A. Shifts to the right with a rise in temperature
    B. Shifts to the left with a decrease in the levels of 2,3-DPG
    C. Is not affected by any change in $PCO_2$
    D. Shifts with pH is known as Bohr effect
    E. If shifted to the left, means oxygen is less readily released to the tissues

36. **Which of the following statements are true:**
    A. $FIo_2$ is the concentration of oxygen in the expired air
    B. $PaO_2$ is significantly affected by $FIo_2$
    C. $PaO_2$ is dependent on the ventilation: Perfusion (V/Q) balance
    D. A $PaO_2$ of <8 kPa reflects a respiratory failure
    E. Normal tidal volume is 1.2 litres

37. **Which of the following statements are true:**
    A. Normal residual volume is 1.2 L
    B. A maximal inhalation after a maximal exhalation gives the vital capacity
    C. Total lung capacity is 2.5 L
    D. Normal $FEV_1$:FVC Ratio is < 0.7
    E. Reduced $FEV_1$ suggests airway obstruction

38. **In ARDS:**
    A. Pulmonary hypotension is a feature
    B. Chest X-ray shows bilateral alveolar oedema
    C. Thoracic compliance is markedly increased
    D. Sepsis and trauma are important causes
    E. Mortality is 5-6%

39. **Which of the following statements are false:**
    A. Frusemide acts on distal collecting tubule
    B. Spironolactone is a loop diuretic
    C. Thiazide diuretics act in the distal tubule
    D. Frusemide causes hyperkalaemia
    E. Amiloride is a potassium sparing diuretic

35. A:T, B:T, C:F, D:T, E:T    36. A:F, B:T, C:T, D:T, E:F
37. A:T, B:T, C:F, D:F, E:T    38. A:F, B:T, C:F, D:T, E:F
39. A:F, B:F, C:T, D:F, E:F

40. Which of the following statements are true about urethral injuries:
   A. May be associated with pelvic fractures
   B. Bleeding and urinary retention are common
   C. Rupture of bulbous urethra is very common
   D. Always require immediate urethral catheterization
   E. Strictures are common sequelae

40. A:T, B:T, C:T, D:F, E:T

## *Answers*

1. **A:F, B:F, C:F, D:T, E:F**
   This patient has been seriously injured following a road traffic accident. His management should be based on the advanced trauma life support (ATLS) guidelines. Airway control with cervical spine immobilisation is the primary step in the management of any trauma patient. The primary survey (initial assessment) should be carried out in the following order:A (*airway*), B (*breathing*), C (*circulation*), D (*disability*) and E (*exposure*).
   ATLS guidelines help in the systematic identification and management of the serious injuries.

      The chances of missing any injury, are also minimised. In this patient, the maintenance of airway and cervical spine immobilisation is the top priority. A referral to a specialist should be made relatively soon but obviously after airway, breathing and circulation have been dealt with efficiently.

2. **A:F, B:F, C:F, D:F, E:T**
   Normal intracranial pressure is about 10 mmHg (136 mm of water). Pressures over 40 mmHg are considered as very high and suggest a poor outcome. A rise in the intracranial pressure causes a decrease in the cerebral perfusion pressure. Following trauma, the intracranial pressure is within normal limits upto a certain stage. When the patient reaches the 'point of decompensation', the intracranial pressure rises expotentially and may cause herniation of the brain.

3. **A:F, B:F, C:T, D:F, E:F**
   The Glasgow Coma Score is very useful in patients with altered levels of consciousness as it gives a fair assessment of the severity of the head injury. Three features are considered:Eye opening (E), Best motor response (M) and Best verbal response (V). The scores obtained from these 3 assessment areas are added together to calculate a final score. The best possible score

is 15 and the minimum score is 3 (GCS of less than 3 is not possible).

| Assessment area | Score |
|---|---|
| Eye opening (E) | |
| - spontaneous | 4 |
| - to speech | 3 |
| - to pain | 2 |
| - to none | 1 |
| Best motor response (M) | |
| - obeys commands | 6 |
| - localises pain | 5 |
| - normal flexion (withdrawal) | 4 |
| - abnormal flexion (decorticate) | 3 |
| - extension (decerebrate) | 2 |
| - none (flaccid) | 1 |
| Verbal response (V) | |
| - orientated | 5 |
| - confused conversation | 4 |
| - inappropriate words | 3 |
| - incomprehensible sounds | 2 |
| - none | 1 |

**4. A:T, B:F, C:T, D:T, E:F**

This patient has lost more than 1500 ml of blood, which is equivalent to more than 30% of his blood volume. His pulse and respiratory rate is expected to increase while the blood pressure and pulse pressure would be low. This patient is extremely unwell. His urine output and mental status are likely to deteriorate if no urgent action is taken. He needs aggressive fluid resuscitation by the crystalloids and blood to compensate for the fluid loss.

It is important to determine the blood loss and note vital parameters (pulse, blood pressure, pulse pressure, respiratory rate, urine output and mental status) in order to assess the severity of the situation following trauma. The patient is graded from class I to class IV based on these findings. The patient can change grades even while being managed in the resuscitation room. Hence, repeated assessment is recommended. The degradation from class II to class III is 'serious'and demands urgent management.

| | Class I | Class II | Class III | Class IV |
|---|---|---|---|---|
| Blood loss (ml) | Up to 750 | 750 to 1500 | 1500 to 2000 | More than 2000 |
| Blood loss (%) blood volume | Up to 15 | 15 to 30 | 30 to 40 | More than 40 |
| Pulse rate | Less than 100 | More than 100 | More than 120 | More than 140 |
| Blood pressure | Normal | Normal | Decreased | Decreased |
| Pulse pressure (mmHg) | Normal or increased | Decreased | Decreased | Decreased |
| Respiratory rate | 14-20 | 20-30 | 30-40 | More than 35 |
| CNS/ mental status | Slightly anxious | Mildly anxious | Anxious and confused | Confused and lethargic |
| Fluid replacement (3:1 rule) | Crystalloids | Crystalloids | Crystalloids and blood | Crystalloids and blood |

NB - The 3:1 rule is based upon the observation that 300 ml of electrolyte solution is required for each 100 ml of blood loss.

5. **A:F, B:F, C:F, D:F, E:F**

Shock may be classified as: hypovolemic, septic, anaphylactic, cardiogenic and neurogenic.

The neurogenic shock, seen after a spinal injury, is produced due to the loss of sympathetic tone. The classical feature is hypotension without tachycardia or cutaneous vasoconstriction. Pulse pressure may remain unchanged in the neurogenic shock. The initial management should primarily be aimed at restoring the volume replacement.

6. **A:T, B:F, C:T, D:F, E:F**
Haemorrhage is the most cause of shock following trauma. Tachycardia and vasoconstriction occur as a direct result of hypovolaemia .

There is volume depletion and a fall in the cardiac output. The correction of class I hypovolaemic shock is satisfactorily achieved by using crystalloids, as a 'fluid challenge'.

The fluid challenge is the initial bolus dose of intravenous fluids given to the patient as a resuscitative measure to treat the shock.

7. **A:F, B:F, C:T, D:T, E:T**

Approximate blood loss:

Fractured humerus and tibia about 500 ml
Fracture pelvis 2000-3000 ml
Fracture femur 1000-2000 ml
These values may vary with the nature of the injury. There may be excessive blood loss (usually, doubled) in compound fractures. A rough estimate of the amount of blood loss can help in assessment and treatment of shock.

8. **A:F, B:T, C:F, D:T, E:F**
Haemorrhage causes hypovolemia which leads to a reduced delivery of oxygen to the peripheral tisssues (shock).

Patients with haemorrhagic shock are usually tachycardic and the peripheries appear cold because of cutaneous vasoconstriction.

The urine output is a sensitive indicator for assessment to the response of treatment of shock. 1 ml/ kg body weight/hour in children and 0.5 ml/kg body weight/hour in an adult, is regarded as a satisfactory measure of good renal blood flow and hence, urinary output. However, a urinary output of 2 ml/kg/hr is necessary, in any child less than one year of age.

An intact airway with adequate ventilatory exchange and oxygenation is the top priority in the management of the haemorrhagic shock. Direct pressure and a pneumatic anti-shock garment (if available) help in the control of bleeding.

A tourniquet should never be used to stop haemorrhage in a trauma patient. Its use can worsen the shock and may lead to limb and life-threatening complications.

9. **A:F, B:T, C:T, D:T, E:T**
   A tension pneumothorax occurs due to the collection of air in the chest wall. It is a potentially life-threatening condition and may result in serious cardiovascular and respiratory effects.

   The most common cause of tension pneumothorax is positive pressure ventilation in a trauma patient. It must be remembered that tension pneumothorax is a clinical diagnosis and radiological confirmation is not necessary. The common features are chest pain, air hunger, respiratory distress, tachycardia, hypotension, tracheal deviation, unilateral absence of breath sounds and features of cyanosis. It can be differentiated with cardiac tamponade on the basis of hyperresonance and absent breath sounds on the affected side. Immediate management is in the form of decompression in the 2nd intercostal space in the mid-clavicular line. The definitive treatment consists of the insertion of a chest drain in the 5th intercostal space.

10. **A:T, B:T, C:T, D:T, E:F**
    Bleeding in the pericardial sac following a penetrating injury leads to 'cardiac tamponade'. This is a serious condition and may cause severe haemodynamic derangement. An elevation in the venous pressure, fall in the arterial pressure and muffled heart sounds constitutes 'Beck's Triad'. These features are useful in

the diagnosis of 'cardiac tamponade'. An exaggeration of the normal fall of systolic blood pressure with spontaneous inspiration may be seen in patients with cardiac tamponade (pulsus parodoxus). 'Kussmaul's sign' represents an elevation in the venous pressure with inspiration during spontaneous breathing. The clinical features of cardiac tamponade are very similar to those of tension pneumothorax but the latter is characterised by absent breath sounds and hyperresonant chest. Cardiac tamponade can be effectively treated by pericardiocentesis (evacuation of blood from the pericardial sac).

11. **A:F, B:T, C:F, D:T, E:T**
The common indications for chest drain insertion are blunt trauma with more than 10% pneumothorax, pneumothorax with patients requiring IPPV or anaesthesia, penetrating trauma with pneumothorax and haemothorax that is visible radiologically. It is important to check the position of the chest drain by a radiological examination of the chest after it has been successfully introduced. The incision for chest drain insertion should always be made on the top of the rib to avoid damage to the intercostal nerves and vessels.

Infection may be introduced as a result of chest drain insertion. Thoracic empyema may follow. Other complications of chest drain insertion are laceration to the lung, liver, etc, damage to the intercostal nerves and vessels, dislodgement of the drain, persistent pneumothorax, subcutaneous emphysema, etc.

12. **A:T, B:F, C:T, D:T, E:F**
A careful rectal examination is necessary after major trauma. It helps in the assessment of the sphincter tone, position of prostate and presence of blood in the rectum.

Tha 'anal tone assessment' is very significant in the spinal cord injuries. A 'high riding' prostate is seen in urethral injuries and, therefore, the position of the prostate should be confirmed. The presence of both, frank and occult, blood can be confirmed by digital examination of the rectum and may be suggestive of a gastrointestinal injury. Certain pelvic fractures can also be detected by examining the rectum.

13. **A:T, B:T, C:T, D:F, E:F**
Involuntary guarding, rebound tenderness, diffuse dullness and bruising are signs of intra-abdominal injury. The presence or absence of bowel sounds does not rule out an intra-abdominal injury and, hence, is of little clinical significance in trauma situations. Bruit and enlarged liver do not contribute to the diagnosis of intra-abdominal trauma.

14. **A:T, B:F, C:F, D:F, E:T**
A profound hypovolaemia, despite resuscitation, may require a laparotomy to identify the source of bleeding. Intra-abdominal bleeding is considered to be an important cause of unexplained hypertension in the trauma patients. Peritonitis, free gas within the abdomen, ruptured diaphragm and gunshot wounds are other important indications for laparotomy. A soft but slightly tender abdomen should be closely monitored but may not necessarily require laparotomy. However, exploration of the abdomen may be considered subsequently, if there are definite signs of intra-abdominal injury.

15. **A:F, B:F, C:T, D:F, E:F**
The cerebral perfusion pressure is of utmost importance in head injuries. It is defined as the mean arterial pressure minus intracranial pressure. It indicates that any rise in the intracranial pressure has a negative effect on the cerebral perfusion pressure. This leads to deficient oxygenation and perfusion to the brain and may cause death.

The head injury is classified as mild (GCS 14-15), moderate (GCS 9-13) and severe (GCS 3-8). This classification system is helpful in determining the severity of the head injury.

Altered level of consciousness, pupillary changes, cranial nerve involvement, periorbital ecchymosis and a leakage of CSF from ears, nose, etc, are signs of a major head trauma. Adequate fluid resuscitation is essential in maintaining the cerebral perfusion pressure and is, therefore, a top priority in the management of head injury patients.

A convex lenticular hyper-dense shadow on the CT strongly suggests an acute extradural haematoma. A subdural haematoma appears as a concave shadow in the CT film. Hyperventilation is useful in a head injury patient because it reduces $PCO_2$ and causes cerebral vasoconstriction. This reduction in the intracranial volume in turn reduces the intracranial pressure. Basal skull fractures are important and serious forms of head injury. Otorrhoea, rhinorrhoea, periorbital cellulitis (racoon eyes), retroauricular ecchymosis (Battle's sign) and 7th nerve palsy are strongly suggestive of a basal skull fracture. However, the diagnosis of this injury can be confirmed only by performing a CT scan and the X-rays are of limited value.

16. **A:F, B:F, C:F, D:T, E:F**
CT scan is useful in the diagnosis of a basal skull fracture. Otorrhoea and rhinorrhoea may occur and this may subsequently lead to 'bacterial meningitis'. The presence of retroauricular ecchymosis is an important feature of basal skull fracture (Battle's sign).

Periorbital cellulitis (also described as 'racoon eyes') combined with other signs of a basal skull fracture like CSF leaks and 7th nerve palsy are important features in the identification of a basal skull fracture.

X-ray probably has no role. Every patient with suspected a basal skull fracture should have a CT for the confirmation of diagnosis.

The role of the prophylactic antibiotics to prevent bacterial meningitis is controversial but nowadays, most neurosurgeons avoid them.

17. **A:F, B:F, C:F, D:T, E:T**

    A hemi section of the cord following injury results in a 'Brown-Séquard syndrome'. It is a very rare injury and is characterised by the involvement of corticospinal tract (ipsilateral motor loss), posterior column (loss of position) and spinal thalamic tract (loss of sensation below the level of injury). The other spinal cord syndromes are classified as anterior and central cord syndromes.

18. **A:F, B:T, C:F, D:T, E:T**

    Crush syndrome is characterised by a 'traumatic rhabdomyolysis'. Myoglobin and other toxic materials are released into the circulation as a result of prolonged compression of the muscle. These toxic materials cause have profound systemic effects. The renal system is particularly affected.

    Various complication like hypovolaemia, metabolic acidosis, hyperkalaemia, hypocalcaemia and disseminated intravascular coagulation, may occur. The urine is dark in colour due to the secretion of myoglobin. The treatment consists of prompt fluid resuscitation in order to prevent renal failure. Osmotic diuresis and alkalisation of the urine may also prove useful.

19. **A:T, B:F, C:F, D:T, E:T**

    Compartment syndrome is characterised by elevation of the pressure in a closed osteofacial compartment. The capillary blood flow is affected if the tissue pressure rises above 35-45 mmHg and this may lead to ischaemic changes to the muscles and nerves locally.

    The intra-compartmental pressure is also related to the systolic blood pressure. This essentially means that if the systolic blood pressure is low, the pressure required to cause compartment syndrome is also low. Pain is the most important symptom and this is exaggerated by passive stretching of the local muscles. Swelling, blistering, alteration of sensation and in the late stages, loss of peripheral pulses may be seen as a result of compartment syndrome. The diagnosis is mainly clinical and may be confirmed by intra-compartmental pressure monitoring. A high index of suspicion is necessary for early diagnosis. External pressure (splints, tight splints, bandage, plaster cast, etc) should be immediately removed and the patient must be closely monitored. Any deterioration in the condition or a persistent elevation of the compartmental pressure, requires urgent and liberal faciotomies.

20. **A:T, B:F, C:F, D:F, E:F**
The radiological evaluation of the cervical spine is essential in a patient with a suspected cervical spine injury. Three sets of X-rays are usually done - AP, lateral and 'open-mouth' neck views. The combination of all 3 views identifies a cervical spine fracture in nearly 95% of cases. In some situations special views like swimmer's views, flexion and extension view, etc may be required. The whole cervical spine should be visualised including the base of the skull and the junction of 7th cervical and 1st thoracic vertebra. These films should be taken in all cases of suspected cervical injury (irrespective of the consciousness levels) once the patient has been stabilised.
A CT scan of the cervical spine is indicated only in cases where clinical and radiological assessment is difficult or the injury needs to be evaluated further.

21. **A:F, B:T, C:T, D:F, E:F**
Chance's fracture is a flexion-distraction injury due to the disruption of the anterior, middle and posterior columns of the lumbar vertebra. It usually occurs in seat-belted patients, and may be associated with serious intra-abdominal and retroperitoneal injuries. It is a serious injury and may require operative stabilisation.
However, the mechanism of a 'burst fracture' is entirely different. The vertebra is subjected to a compressive force rather than a distractive force and the compression causes a shearing force that splits the vertebra into the typical large central and posterior

fragments. This type of injury is commonly seen after a fall from a height.

22. **A:T, B:F, C:T, D:F, E:T**

The circulating volume should be rapidly replaced in a child presenting with shock. An initial bolus of 20 ml/kg body weight is given and this may be repeated on 2 more occasions giving a total of 60 ml/kg body weight.

In children younger than 6 years, interosseous infusion may be considered if percutaneous intravenous access is unsuccessful after 2 attempts.

A urinary output of at least 1 ml/kg body weight per hour is considered to be a healthy response after administration of fluid bolus for shock. The 3:1 rule is applicable to the child as well. Correction of shock by intravenous fluid is based on the body weight and there are different tools available for the assessment of the child's body weight.

23. **A:F, B:T, C:T, D:T, E:T**

Non-accidental injury in a child occurs following an intentional harm by the parents, guardians, etc. The main features of non-accidental injury are absence of correlation between the history and physical findings, prolonged interval between the injury and presentation to the clinicians, repeated trauma treated at different places, inability to comply with the doctor's advice and inconsistency with the history. Multiple subdural haematomas, retinal haemorrhages, perioral injuries, visceral injury, trauma to the genital organs, multiple injuries of different ages, abnormal pattern of injuries such as bites, cigarette burns or burns in unusual areas, etc may be seen.

24. **A:F, B:F, C:T, D:F, E:T**

Ulnar nerve injuries are commonly associated with forearm and wrist lacerations. A weakness of the Adductor pollicis causes over-action of the flexor pollicis longus (from inside).

Inability to grip a piece of paper between the fingers arises from the paralysis of interossei. The lumbricals and interossei flex the metacarpophalangeal joint and extend both proximal and interphalangeal joints. Paralysis of these muscles leads to a 'claw hand' deformity. The interphalangeal joints of the fingers are typically flexed and the metacarpophalangeal joints are extended. Sensory loss in the ulnar nerve lesions is characteristically seen on the medial 1½ fingers.

The ulnar nerve is a branch of the medial cord of the brachial plexus (root value C7,8 and T1). It gives motor branches to flexor carpi ulnaris, medial half of flexor digitorum profundus, palmaris to brevis, medial two lumbricals, all the interossei and both heads of the adductor pollicis. The superficial branch supplies sensation to the ulnar 1½ fingers.

The ulnar nerve is affected in fractures of the pisiform, hook of hamate and may also get compressed in the Guyon's canal.

**25. A:F, B:F, C:T, D:F, E:T**
Explanation same as in Answer 24

**26. A:T, B:F, C:F, D:F, E:T**
The anterior cruciate ligament is an intra-articular ligament of the knee, which is attached in front of the tibial spine anteriorly and over a smooth impression on the lateral condyle of the femur in the intercondular notch posteriorly. Most of the injuries result from sporting activities like netball, skiing, soccer, etc. After injury, the patient usually hears a pop or a snap and develops a haemarthrosis in a few hours. Instability of the knee is a common feature. Lachman, pivot shift and anterior Drawer tests are commonly used to detect instability in the knee. The patient may respond to a course of physiotherapy. Reconstruction of the ligament is considered in a significantly symptomatic knee that has failed to respond to the conservative treatment.

27. **A:F, B:T, C:F, D:T, E:F**
    The Salter Harris classification is used to describe the epiphyseal injuries in children. There are 5 types:
    Type I—fracture line runs along the epiphyseal plate
    Type II—epiphyseal injury is associated with a metaphyseal fragment
    Type III—fracture line extends into the epiphysis
    Type IV—fracture line crosses the epiphyseal plate
    Type V—epiphyseal plate is crushed.
    The prognosis worsens with the increase in the grade of the injury (i.e. Type V has the worst prognosis). The epiphyseal injury may cause a disturbance in the growth of the bones.
    Type II injuries are the most commonly encountered epiphyseal injuries in clinical practice.

28. **A:F, B:F, C:T, D:T, E:T**
    Sepsis is defined as a systemic inflammatory response syndrome following a proven infection. Mortality rates are high and are estimated to be about 16%. The inflammatory reaction is mediated by cytokines, which are released in large amounts following the insult. The activation of the complement system and coagulation pathway causes a variety of systemic changes. There may be alteration in temperature, blood pressure, heart rate and respiratory rate. The myocardial activity is depressed and respiratory alkalosis, renal and liver failure, coagulopathy and increased levels of inflammatory markers may be seen. This is a serious condition and should be aggressively treated by supportive measures like oxygenation, cardiovascular and metabolic stabilisation. Fluids, inotropic support, antibiotic therapy +/- surgical drainage may be indicated.

29. **A:2, B:5: C:7, D:3, E:6**
    The rapid accumulation of more than 1,500 ml of blood in the pleural cavity may lead to a massive pneumothorax. A disruption of the systemic or hilar vessels following penetrating trauma is the most common cause

of this injury. This may lead to hypoxia, hypotension and dullness on percussion with absent breath sounds on the affected side. This condition needs to be managed by aggressive resuscitation with crystalloids, colloids and blood. Defenitive management involves a chest drain and early thoracotomy.

Hypoxia may be caused by large defects of the chest wall resulting from a penetrating wound in the chest. The air is sucked into the chest cavity thus equalising the intra-thoracic and atmospheric pressure. The ventilation is adversely affected. Closure of the wound with occlusive dressings open on one side and closed on three sides allows escape of the air. A chest drain is also required.

A flail chest results from fracture of multiple ribs at two or more places. As a result, the flail segment loses bony continuity with the rest of the thoracic cage. This may result in severe hypoxia and represents an underlying pulmonary contusion. Adequate oxygen and fluid resuscitation, analgesia and close monitoring are essential. Intubation and ventilation may become necessary to increase the arterial content of oxygen.

Mechanical ventilation is the most common cause of tension pneumothorax. This can lead to serious respiratory and haemodynamic disturbances and requires an urgent decompression of the chest cavity by needle thoracentesis followed by insertion of the chest drain. A penetrating injury to the heart may result in cardiac tamponade. This may cause varying degrees of hypoxia, elevation of venous pressure and a marked reduction in the cardiac activity. The clinical signs are similar to those of a 'tension pneumothorax'. However, the chest is hyperresonant with absent breath sounds in tension pneumothorax and these features may help in differentiating between the two conditions. The cardiocentesis followed by thoracotomy is usually necessary.

30. **A:T, B:T, C:F, D:T, E:F**
    The indications for ITU transfer are:

    Conditions requiring intubation
    Respiratory failure requiring ventilation
    Close monitoring of the cardiovascular system (e.g. pulmonary artery floatation catheter (PAFC) and inotropic support)
    Severe metabolic disturbances requiring close observation
    A need for one to one nursing
    A raised urea and/or creatinine may be mildly raised in some patients in the first postoperative day in response to surgical trauma, dehydration, etc. A urea of 30 mmol/l and creatinine of 95 µmol/l without any other abnormality, is certainly not an indication for ICU transfer.
    Similarly, any patient with osteomyelitis secondary to diabetic ulceration in uncomplicated cases can easily be managed as an outpatient or on the wards depending on the status of the wound.

31. **A:F, B:T, C:T, D:F, E:T**
    Prolonged ventilation can result in several systemic complications. The raised intrathoracic pressure causes an elevation in the right atrial pressure which leads to a reduction in the venous return.

    Barotrauma is a known complication after ventilation. The air can escape into the cavities and interstitial tissues.

    Life-threatening complications like tension pneumothorax may be seen following IPPV.

    Rapid correction of hypercapnia in chronic respiratory failure leads to respiratory alkalosis in ventilated patients. This may result in hypoxaemia. The intrathoracic blood volume in the ventilated patients is reduced and vasopressin is secreted in increased amounts from the anterior pituitary gland. This causes increased water retention. Prolonged ventilation may also cause wasting of the respiratory muscles. Nosocomial infections may occur after endotracheal intubation.

32. **A:F, B:F, C:F, D:F, E:F**
The pH is decreased, which suggests acidosis. A reduction in the bicarbonate ion suggests a metabolic cause for the acidosis. This patient is actually hyperventilating and, therefore, has a compensatory respiratory alkalosis.

High white cell and neutrophil counts combined with the metabolic derangements suggest that the patient is extremely unwell with sepsis and requires close monitoring and support in the ITU.

33. **A:F, B:T, C:F, D:T, E:T**
Acute renal failure is characterised by an inability to clear the waste products of metabolism by the kidneys. Common features are drowsiness, confusion, hiccups, twitching, etc. Plasma urea and electrolytes are deranged. Hyperkalaemia, hyponatraemia and metabolic acidosis may be seen. Postoperative renal failure is usually due to acute tubular necrosis and dehydration is an important causative factor. Close monitoring with the use of CVP line and pulmonary artery floatation catheter may become necessary after the onset of acute renal failure. Regular assessment of the urinary output is required for monitoring patients with acute renal failure.

34. **A:T, B:F, C:T, D:T, E:T**
Disseminated intravascular coagulation occurs due to the activation of certain clotting factors mainly thrombin leading to low levels of fibrinogen (consumptive coagulopathy).

Sepsis is considered to be the most important cause for DIC which may result in a generalised bleeding tendency and multi organ failure. The levels of fibrinogen in the blood are reduced, PT and PTT are markedly elevated and thrombocytopenia may be severe.

Treatment of the cause, infusion of fluids, FFP, cryoprecipitate and platelets, if required may improve the condition of the patient.

35. **A:T, B:T, C:F, D:T, E:T**
The oxygen-dissociation curve is a graph that depicts the oxygen saturation of haemoglobin at different pressures of oxygen in the blood. It may shift to the left or to the right depending on oxygen tension. A shift to the left is observed in hyperventilation (low $PCO_2$), alkalosis (high pH), hypothermia and reduced levels of 2, 3DPG (stored blood). In contrast, a shift to the right is seen in acidosis, hypercapnia, anaemia, raised temperature and raised levels of 2, 3DPG.

A shift to the left indicates that the oxygen is less readily released to the tissues while a shift to the right suggests a decreased affinity of haemoglobin for oxygen and thus increased delivery of oxygen to the tissues. The relationship between the shifts of the oxyhaemoglobin curve and pH changes is known as 'Bohr-effect'.

36. **A:F, B:T, C:T, D:T, E:F**
$FIo_2$ is the concentration of oxygen in the inspired air. Oxygen tension in the blood ($PaO_2$) changes significantly with the $FIo_2$. It is also dependent upon the ventilation perfusion ratio.

Respiratory failure is defined as an arterial oxygen tension of less than 8 kPa (60 mmHg). It is further subdivided as

Type I    $PaCO_2 < 6.6$ kPa
Type II   $PaCO_2 > 6.6$ kPa.

Type I respiratory failure is commonly associated with pulmonary and cardiac disease; whereas Type II is linked with disorders of the nervous system and conditions causing alveolar hypoventilation. However, respiratory failure in COPD may be of either types because of ventilation perfusion imbalance. Normal tidal volume is about 500 ml.

37. **A:T, B:T, C:F, D:F, E:T**

The lung function tests are of considerable importance in the overall assessment of the function of the respiratory system. It must be remembered that lung capacity is calculated by the addition of 2 or more volumes. The approximate values for different lung volumes and capacities are as follows:

Tidal volume 500 ml

Residual volume 1.2 L

Expiratory volume 1.3 L

Total lung capacity 6 L

IRV 3 L

FRC 2.5 L.

$FEV_1$ is the volume of air expired in a given time, usually one second, and FVC is the total amount of air expired in litres. $FEV_1$/FVC ratio gives a useful assessment of the degree of impairment in the function of the lung. $FEV_1$/FVC ratio is normally about 0.7 (70%). A value of more than 70% suggests a restrictive lung disease whilst a ratio below 70% indicates obstructive airways disease.

38. **A:F, B:T, C:F, D:T, E:F**

ARDS is the pulmonary manifestation of 'multiple organ failure'. It is characterised by a leakage of fluid from the pulmonary vasculature across the alveolar membrane. Sepsis, trauma, burns, pancreatitis, fat emboli, gastric aspiration, etc are important causes. Hypoxia, reduction in thoracic compliance and pulmonary capillary wedge pressure and bilateral pulmonary infiltrates are the common manifestations of acute respiratory distress syndrome (ARDS). This condition requires circulatory and respiratory support with close monitoring. Treatment of the cause and reduction of risk factors help in the management. Mortality rates are very high ranging from 25-50%.

39. **A:F, B:F, C:T, D:F, E:F**✝

    Commonly used diuretics are classified as loop diuretics, thiazide type diuretics and potassium-sparing diuretics.

    The sites of primary action of these diuretics are different. The loop diuretics, (for example, Frusemide) act on the thick ascending loop of Henlé. Thiazide (e.g. Hydrochlorothiazide) affect the distal tubule and connecting segment. Potassium-sparing diuretics like Spironolactone, Amiloride and Triamterene target the cortical collecting tubule.

    Frusemide causes hypokalaemia and ototoxicity. Thiazides are known to cause hypokalaemia, hypomagnesaemia, hyperglycaemia and thrombocytopenia. GI upsets and hyperkalaemia are common with potassium-sparing diuretics like Amiloride.

40. **A:T, B:T, C:T, D:F, E:T**

    Urethral injuries commonly occur after a fall from a height or on a projecting object, road traffic and cycling accidents, etc. The common features are perineal haematoma, bleeding from the external urinary meatus and urinary retention. Bulbar urethra is most commonly ruptured. Urinary catheterization is indicated in the presence of urinary retention. However, it is contra-indicated, if a rupture of urethra is suspected. A suprapubic catheter may be required in such cases. Stricture and extravasation of urine are the common complications seen after urethral injuries.

# 3

## Neoplasia

1. **Epstein-Barr virus causes:**
   A. Hepatocellular cancer
   B. Adult T-cell lymphoma
   C. Burkitt's lymphoma
   D. Lung cancer
   E. Nasopharyngeal carcinoma

2. **Which of the following statements are true:**
   A. Aflatoxin is an important carcinogenic agent for lung cancer
   B. Ultraviolet radiation is associated with melanoma
   C. Carcinogenesis may involve DNA mutation
   D. All oncogenes produce proteins which limit cell multiplication or transformation
   E. p53 gene is associated with the development of sarcomas

3. **Which of the following statements are true:**
   A. Thyroid cancer is the commonest malignancy in females in the UK
   B. Malignant tumours can not spread through the venous system
   C. Transcoelomic spread is seen in gastric carcinoma and certain ovarian tumours
   D. Cancer surgery may also help in staging the disease
   E. Radical mastectomy is the preffered surgery for all types of breast cancer

4. **The following statements are true:**
   A. Neoadjuvant therapy implies to the treatment instituted before surgery in order to increase its effectiveness
   B. Neoadjuvent therapy is used in rectal cancer for downstaging
   C. Radiotherapy causes oxygen dependent damage
   D. All skin cancers respond very poorly to radiotherapy
   E. Radiotherapy is not indicated in lymph node metastasis from testicular tumours

1. A:F, B:F, C:T, D:F, E:T     2. A:F, B:T, C:T, D:F, E:T
3. A:F, B:F, C:T, D:T, E:F     4. A:T, B:T, C:T, D:F, E:F

5. **The p53 gene is involved in the genesis of:**
   A. Breast cancer
   B. Bladder cancer
   C. Colon cancer
   D. Lung cancer
   E. Malignant melanoma

6. **Radiotherapy is indicated as initial treatment in the following:**
   A. Laryngeal tumours
   B. Early Hodgkin's disease
   C. Carcinoma of upper one-third of oesophagus
   D. As an alternative in patients unfit for surgery
   E. Gliomas of the brainstem

7. **Radiotherapy causes:**
   A. Arm lymphoedema
   B. Gonadal damage
   C. Hypothyroidism
   D. Telangiectasia
   E. No changes in the skin or blood vessels

8. **Cyclophosphamide:**
   A. Is an antimetabolite
   B. Is indicated in melanoma
   C. May cause alopecia and cystitis
   D. Is a cytotoxic agent
   E. Is contraindicated in patients with advanced breast cancer

9. **Which of the following statements are true:**
   A. IL-2 has good antitumour activity and may be used for metastatic renal carcinoma
   B. Methotrexate is useful in breast carcinoma
   C. Doxorubicin is an important antitumour antibiotic
   D. Vincristine binds to the proteins of the cellular microtubules
   E. 5 FU may cause cerebellar symptoms

---

5. A:T, B:T, C:T, D:T, E:F       6. A:T, B:T, C:T, D:T, E:T
7. A:T, B:T, C:T, D:T, E:F       8. A:F, B:F, C:T, D:T, E:F
9. A:T, B:T, C:T, D:T, E:T

10. **Treatment of prostate cancer:**
    A. Diethylstilboestrol
    B. LH-RH agonists
    C. Orchidectomy
    D. Tamoxifen
    E. Flutamide

11. **Tumours which respond poorly to chemotherapy:**
    A. Wilms' tumour
    B. Melanoma
    C. Choriocarcinoma
    D. Ewing's sarcoma
    E. Pancreatic cancer

12. **Tumour markers:**
    A. Have no role in prognosis or relapse
    B. Ideally should have 100% sensitivity and 100% specificity
    C. May be assessed by immunoassay
    D. Are useful in detecting recurrence
    E. Are beneficial in assessing the response to treatment

13. **Ca15-3:**
    A. Levels are very low in advanced Ca breast
    B. Levels are high even in some benign breast conditions
    C. Highly sensitive and specific
    D. If elevated preoperatively suggests poor prognosis
    E. Levels are important in relapse

14. **PSA:**
    A. Elevated if the levels are >1ng/ml
    B. Level is low in BPH and prostitis
    C. Detects capsular invasion better than transurethral ultrasound
    D. Level of >35ng/ml is diagnostic of advanced prostate cancer
    E. High preoperative levels are associated with poor prognosis

---

10. A:T, B:T, C:T, D:F, E:T     11. A:F, B:T, C:F, D:F, E:T
12. A:F, B:T, C:T, D:T, E:T     13. A:F, B:T, C:F, D:T, E:T
14. A:F, B:F, C:F, D:T, E:T

15. **Tamoxifen is:**
    A. An oestrogen agonist
    B. The treatment of choice in young patients with carcinoma of the breast
    C. A cause of vaginal bleeding
    D. More effective in patients with oestrogen positive receptors
    E. Usually given for 15 years in postmenopausal females with breast cancer

16. **Screening for breast cancer:**
    A. Reduces mortality significantly
    B. Consists of screening all women under the age of 50 years
    C. Involves the use of mammography every three years
    D. Leads to overdiagnosis (DCIS) in some cases
    E. Is expensive but cost-effective

17. **Risk factors for Ca breast:**
    A. Early menarche
    B. Family history
    C. Multiparity
    D. Breastfeeding
    E. Oral contraceptives

18. **Paget's disease of the nipple:**
    A. Is characterized by eczema like features around the nipple
    B. Denotes a primary tumour in the bones
    C. Consists of large pale cells with abundant cytoplasm
    D. Is bilateral in 88% of the cases
    E. Commonly causes pruritis

---

15. A:F, B:F, C:T, D:T, E:F       16. A:T, B:F, C:T, D:T, E:T
17. A:T, B:T, C:F, D:F, E:T       18. A:T, B:F, C:T, D:F, E:F

19. **Which of the following statements are true about cancer of the breast:**
    A. White discharge from the nipple is diagnostic of breast cancer
    B. Peau d' orange is seen in advanced breast cancer and is due to cutaneous lymphatic edema
    C. Lymphoedema of the arm is seen following the treatment of breast carcinoma
    D. Radical mastectomy is the operation of choice for lesions < 3 cm in size
    E. Fine needle aspiration cytology may be diagnostic > 90% of the cases

20. **Causes of gynaecomastia:**
    A. Breast abscess
    B. Klinefelter's syndrome
    C. Liver failure
    D. Cimetidine
    E. Puberty

21. **Which of the following statements are true about the colonic cancer:**
    A. Routine 6 monthly screening of all patients above 65 years is done in the United Kingdom
    B. Familial adenomatous polyposis does not require screening of family members until the age of 55 years
    C. Colonoscopy has low sensitivity and specificity
    D. Alteration of bowel habit is uncommon in left sided lesions
    E. Ulcerative colitis is not associated with colonic cancer

22. **Common risk factors for colonic carcinoma:**
    A. Oral contraceptives
    B. Young females
    C. Family history
    D. Familial adenomatous polyposis
    E. p53 gene mutations

---

19. A:F, B:T, C:T, D:F, E:T   20. A:F, B:T, C:T, D:T, E:T
21. A:F, B:F, C:F, D:F, E:F   22. A:F, B:F, C:T, D:T, E:T

23. **Treatment of breast diseases:**

   A. 25-year-old lactating mother with a 4 days history of a painful swelling in the left breast associated with cellulitis and a localised fluctuant area

   B. 40-year-old female with a 3×3 cm swelling in the right breast with a positive cytology and mammography associated with a single enlarged axillary lymph node

   C. A 40-year-old with a 5 cm swelling in the right breast confirmed to be malignant with no clinical evidence of axillary lymph node involvement refusing to have a wide local excision because her mother had recurrence following the same operation. She would rather prefer a more extensive procedure

   D. A 60-year-old female who has recently had surgery for breast cancer and is oestrogen receptor positive

   E. A 38-old-lady with advanced node negative breast cancer having a very poor prognosis refusing surgery

   1. Simple mastectomy
   2. Radiotherapy
   3. Tamoxifen 20 mg for five years
   4. Chemotherapy
   5. Wide local excision with axillary node sampling
   6. Radical mastectomy
   7. Incision and drainage
   8. Enucleation

---

23.  A:7, B:5, C:1, D:3, E:4

24. **Which of the following statements are true about colorectal cancer:**
    A. Duke II stage corresponds to the spread of tumour through the bowel to the serosal surface
    B. A malignant growth in the rectum with a 4 cm of clearance available may be dealt with an anterior resection
    C. Colorectal cancer is the second commonest cause of death from malignant conditions in the UK
    D. Lymph node status has no role in the assessment of prognosis
    E. Most of the growths are adenocarcinomas

25. **5-FU:**
    A. Interferes with DNA synthesis in the malignant cells
    B. Causes bone marrow depression and mucositis
    C. Is not indicated in adjuvant therapy for rectal carcinoma due to high incidence of side effects
    D. Prevents micrometastasis and recurrence after surgery in advanced colorectal cancer
    E. Is a vinca alkaloid

26. **Hodgkin's lymphoma:**
    A. Progressive enlargement of lymph nodes is a prominent feature
    B. Shows poor response to radiotherapy and chemotherapy
    C. Is characterised by the presence of Reed-Sternberg cells
    D. Is associated with Epstein-Barr virus
    E. May be associated with hepatomegaly

27. **Malignant melanoma:**
    A. Is common in black population
    B. Is associated with ultraviolet radiation
    C. Can arise in a pre-existing naevus
    D. Rarely metastasises to extradermal sites
    E. May be associated with satellite lesions

24. A:T, B:T, C:T, D:F, E:T    25. A:T, B:T, C:F, D:T, E:F
26. A:T, B:F, C:T, D:T, E:T    27. A:F, B:T, C:T, D:F, E:T

28. **Which of the following statements are true about malignant melanoma:**
    A. Breslow thickness of 2.5 mm carries a very good prognosis
    B. Clark's level V signifies the involvement of subcutaneous dermis
    C. Amelanotic type has the best prognosis
    D. At least 0.5mm margin is necessary for effective surgical removal
    E. Very commonly seen in prepubertal age group

29. **Signs of a malignant transformation in a mole:**
    A. A reduction in the size
    B. A change in the colour
    C. Itching, crusting and bleeding
    D. A change in the shape
    E. Irregularity and thickening

30. **Which of the following statements are true about gastric carcinoma:**
    A. Pylorus is the commonest site of gastric carcinoma
    B. Helicobacter pylori is associated with gastric cancer
    C. Iron deficiency anaemia is very rarely seen in advanced disease
    D. Trosier's sign indicates lymphatic involvement
    E. Transperitoneal spread is unknown

31. **The following are the features of multiple endocrine neoplasia type II a syndrome:**
    A. Gastrinoma
    B. Parathyroid hyperplasia
    C. Marfanoid facial appearance
    D. Medullary thyroid carcinoma
    E. Pheochromocytoma

---

28. A:F, B:T, C:F, D:F, E:F     29. A:F, B:T, C:T, D:T, E:T
30. A:F, B:T, C:F, D:T, E:F     31. A:F, B:T, C:F, D:T, E:T

## Answers

1. **A:F, B:F, C:T, D:F, E:T**
   Cancer can be caused due to a variety of physical and chemical factors. Some viruses are also known to be associated with specific types of malignancies. Cigarette smoking is related to the lung, laryngeal and bladder cancers. Mesothelioma is common in the asbestos industry; polyvinylcholoride is associated with angiosarcoma of the liver and aflatoxins cause hepatocellular carcinoma.

   Physical factors (e.g. ionising radiation) are known to cause various types of leukaemia and breast cancer. Ultraviolet radiation is associated with melanoma, basal and squamous cell carcinomas of the skin. Examples of oncogenic viruses include human papilloma virus (anogenital cancer), Epstein-Barr virus (Burkitt's lymphoma, nasopharyngeal carcinoma, Hodgkin's disease), Hepatitis B and C viruses (hepatocellular carcinoma), etc.

2. **A:F, B:T, C:T, D:F, E:T**
   Explanation same as above

3. **A:F, B:F, C:T, D:T, E:F**
   Carcinoma of the breast is the commonest cancer (followed by colorectal cancer) in females, in the United Kingdom.

   Malignant tumours can spread directly, through the lymphatic and venous systems. Some cancers spread within the body cavities, e.g. ovarian and gastric malignancies.

   Surgery plays an important role in the diagnosis, staging and treatment of many types of cancers. Radical mastectomy is only reserved for some advanced breast cancers. Nowadays, a more conservative surgical approach is adopted. However the choice of surgery depends upon the nature of the growth, extent of spread and patient's choice.

4. **A:T, B:T, C:T, D:F, E:F**

   Adjuvant therapy implies an extramodality to increase the effectiveness of treatment of cancer. When adjuvant therapy is used preoperatively it is termed as 'neo-adjuvant'. Examples of neoadjuvant therapy are pre-operative radiotherapy for rectal cancer and chemo-radiotherapy for oesophageal and some breast cancers.

   Radiotherapy is very effective in rapidly dividing cells. It is especially used in lymph node metastasis from testicular tumours and is found to be useful for certain types of skin cancers as well.

5. **A:T, B:T, C:T, D:T, E:F**

   The p53 protein is a tumour suppresser gene. It undergoes mutation and causes an expression of an abnormal p53 protein, which is associated with many malignant conditions. Over 50% of bladder, breast, colon and lung cancers are related to the p53 mutations.

6. **A:T, B:T, C:T, D:T, E:T**

   Radiotherapy is used in the following situations:
   i. Radiosensitive tumours such as metastasis from testicular cancers or early Hodgkin's disease
   ii. Sites with better functional or cosmetic results as compared to surgery, for example laryngeal cancer, bladder cancer
   iii. Inoperable tumours, for example pelvic sarcomas, brainstem gliomas, etc.
   iv. In situations where surgery is very risky for example upper or mid oesophageal tumours
   v. Unfit patients, for example, uncontrolled cardio-vascular or respiratory disease.

7. **A:T, B:T, C:T, D:T, E:F**

   Radiotherapy, in large doses, can cause significant damage to the lymphatic vessels. The lymphatic drainage is reduced, which increases the chances of development of oedema in the limb. This is characteristically seen in patients with breast carcinoma who have had postope-rative radiation of their axillary lymph nodes.

The radiation also causes injury to the endothelial cells and connective tissues and leads to impairment of the fine vasculature. This may cause poor wound healing, tissue atrophy, ulceration and telangiectasia. Ovarian cells and spermatogenesis, both, are affected by radiotherapy especially in high doses. Radiotherapy also causes changes in the rapidly dividing cells, e.g. folds of skin, GIT, etc, leading to varying degrees of inflammation, ulceration, desquamation and thinning of the skin, etc. Irradiation to follicular cells, at a later stage, may lead to hypothyroidism in patients.

8. **A:F, B:F, C:T, D:T, E:F**
Cyclophosphamide is a commonly used alkylating agent which causes cytotoxicity of the tumour cells. It is used in breast cancer, small cell lung cancer, Hodgkin's disease, non-Hodgkin's lymphoma, leukaemias and sarcomas. Alopecia, cystitis, nausea and vomiting are common side effects. It acts by bonding to the chemical moeity in the protein and nucleic acids of the cells.

Interleukin-2 is a T-cell growth factor which is responsible for the T-cell mediated immune reaction. It has immunomodulator and anti-tumour properties. It has been found to be effective in metastatic renal cell carcinoma and malignant melanoma.

9. **A:T, B:T, C:T, D:T, E:T**
Methotrexate is an antimetabolite which is active against leukaemia, non-Hodgkin's lymphoma, breast cancer and sarcomas. It may cause plasma toxicity, haematological effects, GI upset, renal and liver dysfunction and mucositis.

Doxorubicin, is an example of an anti-tumour antibiotic. Plasma levels are high and haematological and GI effects are quite common. Other complications like alopecia, cardiomyopathy, etc, may also occur. It is useful in malignancies of the breast, lymphatic system, lung , ovaries, bladder, etc. The action is mediated by its binding effect on the DNA of the tumour cells.

10. **A:T, B:T, C:T, D:F, E:T**

    Androgen ablation, in prostate carcinoma, is carried out by the administration of certain drugs or orchidectomy. Stilboestrol, produces regression of prostate cancer but has significant thrombolytic and cardiovascular complications. LH-RH agonists reduce testosterone levels and, thus, produce castration. An initial rise of pituitary LH production may be seen but eventually testosterone production falls due to high levels of LH-RH and a negative feedback effect on the pituitary for the release of LH. Flutamide and Bicalutamide are pure anti-androgens that may be used for producing androgen ablation in carcinoma of the prostate.

    Tamoxifen is mainly used in carcinoma of the breast. It acts on the oestrogen-receptors by competitive inhibition.

11. **A:F, B:T, C:F, D:F, E:T**

    Advanced tumours that are potentially curable by chemotherapy are acute lymphoblastic leukaemia, germ cell tumours, choriocarcinoma, Ewing's sarcoma, Wilms' tumour and diffuse large cell lymphoma. Tumours that are poorly responsive to chemotherapy are pancreatic cancer, melanoma, soft tissue sarcoma, renal cancer, thyroid cancer and cervical cancer.

    Breast cancer, lymphoma and ovarian tumours are potentially curable if local treatment and adjuvant chemotherapy is given at a suitable stage.

12. **A:F, B:T, C:T, D:T, E:T**

    Tumour marker is a substance present in the body, which can be used for the detection of the presence of a tumour. Common examples are Ca-125 (ovarian tumour), carcinoembryonic antigen - CEA (colonic carcinoma), prostatic surface antigen - PSA (prostate cancer), Ca15-3 (breast cancer), etc. They are very useful in the screening and diagnosis of the condition. They also help in monitoring the therapy and in indicating prognosis and relapse.

Tumour markers can be detected by immunoassay or immuno histiochemistry. An ideal tumour marker should have 100% sensitivity and specificity.

13. **A:F, B:T, C:F, D:T, E:T**
Ca15-3 is an important tumour marker for the detection of breast cancer, especially in the advanced stage. However, 2-20% of patients with benign breast disease also show elevated levels of this tumour marker. Hence, it lacks specificity and sensitivity. High preoperative levels are suggestive of a poor prognosis and they also indicate a high chance of relapse. Ca15-3 levels may fall in response to the systemic therapy but this effect is very variable between patients. Hence, this tumour marker is not considered a reliable method for assessing response to treatment.

14. **A:F, B:F, C:F, D:T, E:T**
A great majority of patients with prostatic carcinoma have elevated levels of prostatic surface antigen, PSA (more than 4 ng/ml). It is also found to be elevated in benign prostate conditions like BPH, prostitis, prostatic infarction, urinary retention, instrumentation, etc.
Transurethral ultrasound is preferred to PSA for the detection of capsular invasion in carcinoma of the prostate.
Elevated levels of PSA can be used in the assessment of bony metastasis. High preoperative levels suggest a poor prognosis. A level of more than 35 ng/ml is diagnostic of advanced prostatic cancer. A fall in the level of the PSA to the normal range subsequent to hormonal ablation is a good prognostic sign.

15. **A:F, B:F, C:T, D:T, E:F**
Tamoxifen, is a commonly used drug for the treatment of carcinoma of the breast, especially in postmenopausal females with oestrogen positive receptor status. It is an oestrogen antagonist and is found to be effective in both oestrogen positive and oestrogen negative individuals.

However, the effect in the former group is much pronounced and plays a significant role in preventing recurrence. The side effects of this drug are vaginal bleeding, nausea, weight gain, hot flushes and rarely, endometrial carcinoma. The usual regime of treatment is 20 mg for a period of about 5 years.

16. **A:T, B:F, C:T, D:T, E:T**
Screening for breast cancer significantly reduces the risk of mortality by early identification of the disease. About 20% of tumours, not clinically palpable, are detected by screening. Following publication of the Forest Report in 1987, the UK government has launched a National Breast Screening Programme which involves a 3 yearly mammographic assessment of all females between the ages of 50 to 64 years. Some studies are in progress to extend the upper age limit from 64 to 70. Early detection including screening helps in avoiding expensive and complicated treatment of advanced breast cancer and provides reassurance to the patients. However, in some cases, it may cause unnecessary anxiety and may lead to over-diagnosis of Ca breast (DCIS).

17. **A:T, B:T, C:F, D:F, E:T**
Common risk factors for carcinoma of the breast are early menarche, a history of breast cancer in the family, nulliparity, use of oral contraceptives, early menopause, obesity, etc. These factors increase the risk of developing breast cancer. However, breast cancer is less likely to develop in multiparous females, at young age pregnancy and early menopause.

18. **A:T, B:F, C:T, D:F, E:F**
Paget's disease usually represents an underlying breast carcinoma. This eczematous-like condition of the nipple and areola, needs to be differentiated from true eczema which is due to atopy. Features like pruritus and vesicular eruptions on both nipples are commonly seen in eczema, whilst they are absent in Paget's disease due

to an underlying ductal carcinoma. Microscopically, the cells involved in Paget's disease possess abundant cytoplasm in the malpighian layer of the epidermis and are large in size.

19. **A:F, B:T, C:T, D:F, E:T**
Discharge from the nipple can give a clue to the diagnosis:
White  - lactating breast
Yellow - abscess
Green  - duct ectasia
Red (blood) - ductal papilloma or carcinoma

Peau d'orange represents cutaneous oedema due to lymphatic obstruction. It is a sign of advanced malignancy in the breast. Massive lymphoedema of the arm may result following radical axillary dissection of radiotherapy or both. This, probably, occurs due to the lymphatic and venous blockage following surgery or radiation. Wide local excision combined with axillary node sampling is the preferred method of treatment for early and small malignant lesions of the breast. However, mastectomy, radiotherapy, adjuvant systemic therapy by Tamoxifen and other drugs may become necessary depending upon the stage of the disease, size of the tumour, patient's characteristics and preferences. Fine needle aspiration cytology of a palpable swelling may have a diagnostic accuracy of more than 90% and is commonly used in the assessment of breast lesions in addition to the clinical examination and mammography ('triple assessment').

It is important to note that the treatment of breast cancer, in general, is very controversial and, therefore, different surgeons may adopt different approaches, especially in relation to axillary node sampling and dissection.

20. **A:F, B:T, C:T, D:T, E:T**
Gynaecomastia refers to the enlargement of the male breast. The causes may be idiopathic, Klinefelter's

syndrome, liver failure, drugs like Digoxin, Cimetidine, Spironolactone, puberty old age, endocrine causes such as hypothyroidism or hypogonadism, etc.

21. **A:F, B:F, C:F, D:F, E:F**
Routine colonoscopic screening is not recommended for colorectal carcinoma as it is not cost-effective and patient compliance is low. The family members of individuals suffering from familial adenomatous polyposis, however, require regular screening.

It must be remembered that familial adenomatous polyposis is a disease of young age and usually manifests before the age of 20. If there are no polyps at 20 years of age, screening should continue with 🦠 yearly examination up to the age of 50. A genetic polyp is unlikely. Colonoscopy has a very high sensitivity and specificity for detecting colonic cancer. The common features of carcinoma of the left side of the colon are pain, alteration of bowel habit, palpable lump, distension along with other systemic features of anorexia, weight loss, etc. The overall risk for the development of malignancy following ulcerative colitis is about 3.5%. However, after 20 years of the disease the risk may increase up to 20%. All patients with long-standing ulcerative colitis (more than 10 years) should have regular colonoscopy for an early detection of malignant transformation.

22. **A:F, B:F, C:T, D:T, E:T**
The common risk factors for colonic carcinoma are age (more common in patients over 60 years of age), a low fibre diet, smoking, familial adenomatous polyposis, ulcerative colitis, family history (more common in first degree relatives), hereditary non-polyposis colorectal cancer and p53 gene mutations.

23. **A:7, B:5, C:1, D:3, E:4**
   - This patient most likely has a breast abscess because there is a short history, the swelling is painful,

fluctuant and associated with cellulitis. Definitive treatment is incision and drainage.

- This lady has a breast cancer in its early stages and would therefore be suitable for a wide local excision and axillary node sampling.
- This patient is probably a candidate for simple mastectomy due to the large size of the swelling and her own preference. Axillary dissection may or may not be required.
- This scenario refers to a postmenopausal female who is 'oestrogen receptive sensitive' and would therefore benefit from a course of Tamoxifen (usually given as 20 mg daily for 5 years).
- This young lady who has a very poor prognosis should receive chemotherapy (Cyclophosphamide, Methotrexate and 5-fluorouracil) for her advanced breast cancer.

It is important to note that there is no universal agreement regarding the treatment of breast cancer and, therefore, there may be slight variations in the management of the above-mentioned conditions, especially in relation to the axillary node dissection and the choice of the procedure.

24. **A:T, B:T, C:T, D:F, E:T**
Most of the malignant colorectal growths are adenocarcinomas. Duke's classification is useful in staging the disease and suggesting the prognosis.
- Duke's A—tumour is confined to the wall of the bowel but has not spread outside the muscularis propria
- Duke's B—tumour has spread through the bowel wall to the serosal surface
- Duke's C—there is lymph node involvement ($C_1$ - local lymph nodes and $C_2$ -mesenteric nodes)
- Duke's D—distant metastasis.

Colorectal cancer is the second (after Ca bronchus) commonest cause of death from malignant diseases in the United Kingdom. The lymph node status plays a significant role in assessing the prognosis. The prognosis is poor if more than four lymph nodes are involved by the secondary carcinoma. Any tumour less than 15 cm from the anal verge should have at least 2 cm of clearance available for being suitable for an anterior resection. However, if it is very distal and a margin of at least 2 cm of normal bowel is not available (for example, large tumours in the distal third of the rectum) combined abdominal and perineal excision may be carried out.

25. **A:T, B:T, C:F, D:T, E:F**
5-Fluorouracil is an antimetabolite which interferes with DNA synthesis in the malignant cells. It is used as an adjuvant therapy in advanced colorectal cancer. It is known to reduce the incidence of metastasis and can prolong survival. Important side effects are myelodepression, mucositis and rarely, cerebellar syndrome.

26. **A:T, B:F, C:T, D:T, E:T**
Hodgkin's lymphoma is a malignant condition leading to a progressive enlargement of the lymph nodes. Exact aetiology is not known but the Epstein-Barr virus has been found in the neoplastic cells and also in the serum of patients. It may be associated with fever, weight loss, night sweats, hepatic and splenic enlargement.

Four subtypes are described: lymphocyte predominant, mixed cellularity, nodular sclerosing and lymphocyte depleted.

Staging is done to assess the extent of the disease. Stages I to IV are described. It responds well to radiotherapy in the initial stages. Chemotherapy is reserved for advanced stages (II to IV).

Lymphocyte predominant and nodular sclerosing types have a better prognosis than other subtypes.

27. **A:F, B:T, C:T, D:F, E:T**
Malignant melanoma is a neoplasm of the epidermal melanocytes. It has a high incidence in Caucasians and

is closely related to ultraviolet radiation. It is, therefore, more common in certain geographical areas, e.g. Australia.

Pre-existing naevus can undergo malignant change and transform into a malignant melanoma. It metastasises by local extension, lymphatics and bloodstream. Local satellite lesions are produced following lymphatic permeation and may lead to secondary lymphoedema. Visceral and multiple lymphatic metastases may be seen in the advanced stages.

28. **A:F, B:T, C:F, D:F, E:F**
Malignant melanoma occurs due to a malignant transformation in the epidermal melanocytes. It may be of 5 clinical types: lentigo maligna, superficial spreading, nodular, acral lentiginous and amelanotic. Lentigo maligna melanoma has the best prognosis while the amelanotic type carries a very poor prognosis. The superficial spreading melanomas are the most commonly seen malignant melanomas. The edge of the lesion is irregular and it has a characteristic variegated pattern. Clark's levels and Breslow's grading can assess the depth of invasion of the melanoma.

| Breslow thickness | 5 years survival (%) | Clearance required |
|---|---|---|
| Less than 0.76 mm | More than 95 | 1 cm |
| 0.76-1.5 mm | 85 | 2 cm |
| More than 1.5 mm | Less than 75 | 3 cm |

**Clark staging:**
Stage I - epidermal involvement
Stage II - papillary dermis involvement
Stage III - interface of papillary and reticular dermis involved
Stage IV - involvement of reticular dermis
Stage V - involvement of subcutaneous tissue.

The prognosis becomes worse with increase in the depth of the lesion. At least a 2 cm margin is required for complete excision of a suspicious lesion. Malignant melanoma is rarely seen in the prepubertal age group. It is known to spread by local extension and through the lymphatic and bloodstream. It produces local satellite lesions via the lymphatic system. In advanced cases, lungs, liver, brain, skin and rarely bones may show secondary deposits. Treatment is mainly surgical and requires sufficient clearance.

29. **A:F, B:T, C:T, D:T, E:T**
A malignant transformation in a mole should be suspected if there is a change in size, shape, colour, margins or thickness of the lesion. Crusting or bleeding, sensory changes in the form of increased itching and signs of inflammation again go in favour of malignancy. A high index of suspicion should be kept because early diagnosis and treatment can result in a very good prognosis of this malignant lesion.

30. **A:F, B:T, C:F, D:T, E:F**
Gastric carcinoma is multifactorial in origin. *H. pylori* infection, gastritis, gastric ulcer, pernicious anaemia and gastric atrophy, cigarette smoking, dietary habits, environmental factors, etc. are considered to be the risk factors. The commonest site for gastric malignancy is the antrum and almost all cancers are adenocarcinomas. Microscopically, signet-ring cells containing mucin are characteristic of the gastric malignancy. Iron deficiency anaemia is very common in advanced stages because the cancer tends to bleed heavily. Obstructive features may also be seen in addition to dyspepsia, weight loss, early satiety, bloating, distension, etc. Thrombophlebitis secondary to gastric carcinoma is referred to as 'Trousseau's sign'; while 'Trosier's sign' indicates an enlargement of the supraclavicular lymph node.

Transperitoneal spread is common in this malignant condition. It indicates advanced disease. Krukenberg's tumour, is the classical example, indicating the spread to the ovary through the trans-coelomic route. Secondary deposit appearing at the umbilicus through the abdominal cavity is referred to as 'Sister Joseph's nodule'.

Some form of gastrectomy may be required in the early disease. Systemic adjuvant chemotherapy has not shown encouraging results. However, chemotherapy may be considered in advanced cases.

31. **A:F, B:T, C:F, D:T, E:T**

Multiple endocrine neoplasia syndrome is a disorder characterised by multiple endocrine adenomas associated with APUD cells (amine precursor uptake and decarboxylation). The disorder is autosomal dominant and runs in families. It is of 3 types—type I, type II A and type II B. Type I is the most common variant and is associated with pituitary and pancreatic islet cell adenomas along with parathyroid hyperplasia or adenomas. MEN type II A includes medullary thyroid carcinoma, pheochromocytoma and parathyroid hypoplasia. MEN type II B consists of features of MEN type II A and some additional neurological components. Mucosal neuromas and a characteristic Marfanoid facial appearance along with megacolon and ganglioneuromas may also be seen.

# 4

## Haemopoietic and Lymphoreticular Disorders

1. Causes of thrombocytopenia:
   A. DIC
   B. Hypersplenism
   C. DVT
   D. CHF
   E. SLE

2. Which of the following statements are true about clotting:
   A. Normal activated partial thromboplastin time (APTT) is 3-5 minutes
   B. APTT measures the extrinsic pathway
   C. Normal prothrombin time is 13-15 seconds
   D. Thrombin time is increased in heparin therapy
   E. Deficiencies of fibrinogen can be detected by thrombin time

3. von Willebrand's disease:
   A. May be autosomal dominant
   B. Is characterised by excessive platelet adherence
   C. Commonest presentation is haemarthrosis
   D. Bleeding time is markedly decreased
   E. Factor VIII concentrates are used in the treatment

4. Which of the following statements are true about congenital bleeding disorders:
   A. Protein C causes increased production of fibrin
   B. Deficiency of antithrombin III is a risk factor for venous thrombosis
   C. Haemophilia A is commonly known as Christmas disease
   D. Haemophilia A is usually an X-linked disorder
   E. Haemarthrosis may be seen in haemophilia

5. Causes of lymphoedema:
   A. Radiotherapy to axilla
   B. Postoperative
   C. Milroy's disease
   D. Malaria
   E. Fracture neck of femur

---

1. A:T, B:T, C:F, D:F, E:T      2. A:F, B:F, C:T, D:T, E:T
3. A:T, B:F, C:F, D:F, E:T      4. A:F, B:T, C:F, D:T, E:T
5. A:T, B:T, C:T, D:F, E:F

6. **Lymph node:**
   A. Metastasis is an uncommon feature in the papillary carcinoma of thyroid
   B. Consists of T-cells arranged around a central arteriole
   C. Irradiation is contraindicated in node positive breast cancer
   D. Involvement may be seen in tuberculosis
   E. Involvement is used in the staging of Hodgkin's lymphoma

7. **Common side effects of steroids:**
   A. Inflammation           B. Diabetes
   C. Osteosclerosis         D. Cushing's disease
   E. Psychosis

8. **Cyclosporin:**
   A. Is a commonly used drug in immunosuppression
   B. Causes gingival hypertrophy
   C. Can suppress both antibody production and cell mediated immunity
   D. Causes dose dependent renal side effects
   E. Is a proton pump inhibitor

9. **In splenectomy:**
   A. There is a sudden fall in the white cell and platelet count
   B. Ligation of short gastric vessels is a contraindication
   C. There is an increased risk of postoperative septicaemia
   D. OPSI is a major concern
   E. Oral antibiotic prophylaxis is indicated

10. **Which of the following statements are true:**
    A. Cyclosporin acts by blocking IL-2 gene transcription
    B. HLA class I antigens are HLA-DR, HLA-DP, HLA-DQ
    C. The risk of developing non-Hodgkin's lymphoma is very high after transplantation
    D. Hyperacute rejection occurs 18 months after transplantation
    E. CD-4 cells are important in graft rejection

---

6. A:F, B:F, C:F, D:T, E:T      7. A:F, B:T, C:F, D:T, E:T
8. A:T, B:T, C:T, D:T, E:F      9. A:F, B:F, C:T, D:T, E:T
10. A:T, B:F, C:T, D:F, E:T

## Answers

1. **A:T, B:T, C:F, D:F, E:T**
   Causes of thrombocytopenia are as follows:
   Marrow failure, megaloblastosis, etc → reduced production
   ITP, DIC, SLE, lymphoma, etc → reduced survival of platelets
   Heparin induced (in a small percentage of cases) → platelet aggregation.

2. **A:F, B:F, C:T, D:T, E:T**
   Normal activated partial thromboplastin time—30 to 40 seconds; measures the intrinsic as well as the common pathway.
   Normal prothrombin time—11 to 13 seconds; used in the measurement of extrinsic system
   (Factor VII and tissue factor activate factor X, which helps in the formation of fibrin by the activation of thrombin).
   Heparin treatment increases the thrombin time which is normally 14 to 16 seconds.

3. **A:T, B:F, C:F, D:F, E:T**
   von Willebrand's disease is the most common congenital bleeding disorder and is usually inherited as an autosomal dominant condition. It is characterised by severe bleeding tendencies. Haemorrhage may be seen postoperatively or following trauma. Mucosal bleeds and menorrhagia are also common. Haemarthrosis or muscle haematomas are very rarely seen. The clotting mechanism is deranged and this may lead to an increase in the bleeding time. Factor VIII concentrates are usually used for the management of this condition.

4. **A:F, B:T, C:F, D:T, E:T**
   The congenital deficiencies of protein C and protein S lead to the development of bleeding tendencies by causing a reduction in the formation of fibrin. Antithrombin III inactivates many clotting factors and

may increase the risk of venous thrombosis. Haemophilia is an X-linked recessive disorder. The common types are, haemophilia A and haemophilia B (also known as Christmas disease). Haemophilia is characterised by spontaneous haemorrhages into the soft tissues, muscles and large joints. Treatment consists of the administration of the appropriate factor (haemophilia A—deficiency of factor VIII, haemophilia B—deficiency of factor IX).

5. **A:T, B:T, C:T, D:F, E:F**
Lymphoedema is characterised by a collection of lymph in the subcutaneous tissues following obstruction to the lymphatic flow. It may be caused by the congenital malformations of the lymphatic system, surgical excision and/or irradiation of lymph nodes and lymphatics, filariasis, etc. Many cases of lymphoedema are idio-pathic. Application of external pneumatic compression is the most common mode of treatment for lympho-edema. Surgical therapy has been attempted with variable results.

6. **A:F, B:F, C:F, D:T, E:T**
A typical lymph node consists of a thin fibrous capsule and lymphoid follicles containing germinal centres that are arranged around the periphery. These follicles are composed of B lymphoid cells. The interfollicular areas and the medulla consist of B-lymphoid cells. Other important structures are afferent any efferent lymphatics, outer cortex and inner medulla, subcapsular and medullary sinuses and trabeculae.

The enlargement of regional lymph nodes is a common feature in papillary carcinoma of the thyroid.

Prophylactic radiation of the lymph nodes may be required in breast cancer, especially in a node positive tumour.

The spread to the lymph nodes is useful in assessing the extent of the disease in Hodgkin's and non-Hodgkin's lymphoma. The disease is classified into stages I to IV, depending upon the group of lymph nodes involved.

Lymphadenopathy may also be seen in tuberculosis, sarcoidosis, Crohn's disease, malignancy, cat-scratch disease, lymphogranuloma venereum, etc. The examination of lymph nodes is of vital importance especially in cases of infection and malignancy.

7. **A:F, B:T, C:F, D:T, E:T**
Steroids are used for a variety of medical and surgical conditions. They are known to improve the prognosis by controlling the severity and progress of the disease. However, they should be used with caution especially when administered on a long-term basis. The common side effects are *gastrointestinal*—dyspepsia, peptic ulceration, pancreatitis, etc, *musculoskeletal*—myopathy, osteoporosis, avascular necrosis, etc, *endocrine*—Cushing's syndrome, hirsutism, weight gain, menstrual irregularities, etc, *neuropathic*—psychological disturbances, depression, insomnia, etc, *Ophthalmic*—glaucoma, cataracts, etc, *skin disorders*, etc.

8. **A:T, B:T, C:T, D:T, E:F**
Cyclosporin is the most commonly used drug for immunosuppression in organ transplantation. It is known to cause nephrotoxicity, hepatotoxicity, tremors, convulsions, gingival hypertrophy, haematological abnormalities, raised blood pressure, skin infections, malignant changes, etc. It suppresses, both, humeral and cell mediated immunity. Its administration should be regularly monitored due to serious side effects, especially in relation to kidneys.

9. **A:F, B:F, C:T, D:T, E:T**
Splenectomy may be indicated in the following situations: Trauma, radical gastrectomy, hypersplenism, spherocytosis, varicocele surgery and rarely, Hodgkin's lymphoma.

The short gastric vessels are ligated and divided before the spleen is removed.

The common complications of splenectomy are haemorrhage, gastric dilatation, atelectasis, injury to viscera - pancreas, stomach, etc, and postsplenectomy infections. Splenectomy is usually followed by a marked rise in the white cell and platelet count leading to a risk of thrombosis and anticoagulation is usually necessary.

The most important complication related to splenectomy is infection. Pneumococcal antitoxin (Pneumovax) is advised 2 weeks preoperatively to prevent opportunistic postsplenectomy infection (OPSI). There is also an increased risk of *Streptococcus pneumoniae*, *Neisseria meningitidis*, and *Haemophilus influenzae* infections. Prophylactic oral antibiotics (Penicillin) are advised up to 2 years following splenectomy. Any infection in splenectomy patients should be immediately treated. Special advice and antibiotics are necessary when the patient visits any country where tropical infections are common, for example, malaria.

10. **A:T, B:F, C:T, D:F, E:T**
    Cyclosporin is the most commonly used drug for immunosuppressive therapy during transplantation.

    CD4 T-cells play a significant role in the graft rejection process by the activation of cytokines. Histocompatibility Leukocyte antigens (HLA) are derived from the genes located on chromosome number 6 collectively known as major histocompatibility complex (MHC). There are 2 groups of HLA antigens—class I and class II. HLA class I comprises HLA, HLAB and HLAC. HLA class II antigens are HLADR, HLADP and HLADQ. It is very important to match the donor and recipient histocompatibility antigens in renal transplantation in order to avoid the risk of graft rejection. There are 3 types of grafts rejections—hyper-acute rejection (occurs immediately), acute rejection (occurs in the first 6 months) and chronic rejection (occurs a few months and years after the transplantation). The hyperacute rejection usually takes place due to the presence of cytotoxic antibodies against the HLA class I antigen in the recipient's serum. The administration of immunosuppressive therapy may lead to the development of serious malignant diseases, e.g. non-Hodgkin's lymphoma, skin cancer, Kaposi's sarcoma, etc. This is commonly seen in malignancies, which have a viral aetiology. Fifty percent of transplantations are likely to develop skin cancer in about 20 years. The overall risk of the development of non-Hodgkin's lymphoma is quite high after immunosuppression. Kaposi's sarcoma, although very uncommon, is 300 times more likely to occur in transplant patients.

# 5

---

# Evaluation of Surgery and General Topics

1. The following features are necessary for diagnosing brainstem death:
   A. Absent pupillary reflex
   B. Positive gag reflex
   C. Absent caloric response
   D. Spontaneous breathing when disconnected from the ventilator
   E. Absent corneal reflex

2. Clinical audit:
   A. Is the same as research and involves a hypothesis
   B. Is a process aimed at improvement in the delivery of the health care to the patients
   C. Structure, process and outcome are important components
   D. Is an important part of the surgical training and recommended by the Royal College of Surgeons
   E. Should always be performed by the nurses and the paramedical staff only

3. Which of the following statements are true about consent in the UK:
   A. Valid if given and signed by anybody above 16 years of age with a sound mind
   B. Valid if given and signed by a 14 year old child who is able to understand the pros and cons of the procedure under consideration
   C. Not necessary in malignant diseases
   D. The surgeon may proceed to operate on a patient in serious conditions like septic arthritis even if the patient refuses surgery
   E. Invalid if given by the neighbour

---

1. A:T, B:F, C:T, D:F, E:T     2. A:F, B:T, C:T, D:T, E:F
3. A:T, B:T, C:F, D:T, E:T

4. **P-value:**
   A. Is used in finding the statistical significance
   B. Is not a reliable parameter in clinical research
   C. Is used to test the null hypothesis
   D. Automatically gives the average number of cases involved
   E. Can be calculated by using a software

5. **Which of the following statements are true:**
   A. Randomised controlled trial involves a control group
   B. Chi-square test may be used for statistical analysis
   C. Clinical trial of a new drug in the United Kingdom requires the approval of the Ethics Committee
   D. Type II errors are related to small sample size
   E. A retrospective study is more reliable than a prospective randomised controlled double blinded study

6. **Which of the following statements are false:**
   A. Sensitivity is a measure of all true positive cases
   B. Specificity defines how reliably the test is negative in health
   C. Mammography should not be used for breast cancer occurring in families
   D. Screening test doesn't have to be cost effective
   E. A good test is never highly specific or sensitive

7. **Which of the following statements are true:**
   A. Median refers to the middle value with equal number of observations above and below
   B. Standard deviation gives the extent of dispersion from the mean
   C. Symmetrical distribution is also known as gaussian distribution
   D. Mode is the smallest or greatest value in a distribution
   E. Mean is the sum of observations divided by the number of observations

---

4. A:T, B:F, C:T, D:F, E:T    5. A:T, B:T, C:T, D:T, E:F
6. A:T, B:T, C:F, D:F, E:F    7. A:T, B:T, C:T, D:F, E:T

8. **The audit cycle consists of:**
   - **A.** A standard practice
   - **B.** Observation
   - **C.** Comparison of practice with the standard practice
   - **D.** Implementing a change
   - **E.** Experiments to test a hypothesis

---

8. A:T, B:T, C:T, D:T, E:F

## Answers

1. **A:T, B:F, C:T, D:F, E:T**

   Absence of cranial nerve reflexes — pupillary reflex, corneal reflex, gag reflex and caloric response is an important feature in the diagnosis of death. The other important signs are the absence of motor response and spontaneous respiration when disconnected from a ventilator.

   According to the UK brain death criteria, there should be an absence of drug intoxification, hypothermia, hypoglycaemia, acidosis and urea and electrolyte imbalance. Two clinicians with more than 5 years of clinical experience must diagnose brainstem death and the examination of the patient should be carried out on 2 different occasions. The diagnosis of brain death is of special consideration in organ donation (kidney, liver, cornea, heart or lungs) and this should be discussed at length with the patient's relatives.

2. **A:F, B:T, C:T, D:T, E:F**

   Audit is a process of evaluation of any practice in health care in order to improve the delivery of health services to the community. Audit involves comparison with a standard practice and is usually, described as a loop or a cycle. It differs from research as it does not involve any experiments or trials and no hypothesis is proposed.

   Audit is an important part of postgraduate medical training. It is recognized as an important component of surgical training by all the Royal Colleges.

3. **A:T, B:T, C:F, D:T, E:T**

   In the United Kingdom, a valid consent can be given by anybody above the age of 16 years who is able to understand the pros and cons of the procedure under consideration. In some cases, children of 13 years or above may be allowed to give consent.

   However, the child should be encouraged to discuss the proposed treatment with his parents before he independently gives his consent. The issues related to consent are very vital and should be treated with due consideration. The consent form is not a legal proof of consent but it only indicates that an attempt has been made to obtain an informed consent. Nobody can give an informed consent on behalf of an adult patient. However, in some cases, when the patient is in a serious condition (e.g. unconsciousness), the surgeon may proceed to institute life and or limb saving measures, without consent, in the best interest of the patient.

4. **A:T, B:F, C:T, D:F, E:T**
   The determination of P-value helps to test the null hypothesis. It is an important tool for statistical analysis in clinical research. It helps in the analysis of the results and may be calculated easily by entering data into the computer. Various softwares, e.g. SPSS, are available to calculate the P-value in any clinical study.

5. **A:T, B:T, C:T, D:T, E:F**
   Various types of studies can be conducted in research. The common examples are randomised control, randomised, longitudinal, observational, etc. A retrospective study means analysis of data from past events. This may introduce a lot of bias in the study and may lead to false results. However, a prospective collection of data with randomisation and blinding (single blind or double blind) produces the best results.
   A randomised control study involves one normal and another experimental group. The normal or the control group helps in comparison.
   Sample size is an important modality in any study and 2 types of errors have been described in relation to the sample size. Type 1 errors relate to false positive results, or in other words the benefits are perceived when really there is none. In type 2 errors, the benefit is missed because the study has small numbers (false negative).

6. **A:T, B:T, C:F, D:F, E:F**

   Mammography is an important investigation used for the screening of the female population for breast cancer. A good screening test should be highly specific, sensitive, cost-effective and must have good patient compliance.

7. **A:T, B:T, C:T, D:F, E:T**

   The mean, mode and median are important parameters in the assessment of the numerical data.

   'Median' refers to the middle value with equal numbers of observations above and below. The 'mode' is the value of the variable at which the frequency curve reaches a peak. It can be unimodal or bimodal and usually lies in the middle of the gaussian curve, i.e. between the two extremes of the distribution. The 'mean' or 'average' is the sum of the observations divided by the number of observations. It gives some indication of the general level of a series of measurements.

8. **A:T, B:T, C:T, D:T, E:F**

   Audit is a dynamic process aimed at achieving an improvement in the quality of the delivery of health care. It is usually described as a cycle or a loop. This audit cycle consists of acceptance of a standard practice, making observations to check if the standard practice is being followed and when instituting changes observations reveal a difference from the standard practice. After a certain period of time when these adjustments or changes have been made, the observations are recorded again and compared with the standard practice. If the subsequent results show that the standards have been met, the audit cycle is completed or the loop is 'closed'. However, if the satisfactory results are not achieved, continuous changes are made. The practice is then re-audited.

# Self-assessment

# Self-assessment

The following two sections consist of two papers, which the readers are advised to attempt only when they find themselves 'ready' for the MRCS examination. Each section consists of sixty stems with multiple choices (300 questions) and is based on the format of the actual examination. In fact, several questions in these papers have appeared in the MRCS examinations of the various Royal Colleges in different forms.

Sit in a quite room with a pencil and blank answer sheet and start attempting these questions aiming to finish each paper within 2 hours. Remember, this is an opportunity to test yourself in an 'exam-like'situation, so stick to the guidelines given above. You may use the following 'scoring criteria' to judge where you stand after your first attempt:

More than 80%: Good. preparation. Probably ready to appear in the exam

50-80%: Some more reading essential

30-50%: Extensive reading and revision required

Less than 30%: Not ready for examination at all.

Need advise, guidance and preparation before proceeding any further

Please don't be misled (or dis-heartened) by your scores. They will only give a rough assessment of your preparation. Good luck!

## PAPER I

*(Answer the following questions as True or False; Time Allowed:120 minutes)*

1. **Complications of tracheostomy:**
   A. Tracheal stenosis
   B. Infection
   C. Aortic rupture
   D. Tracheo-oesophageal fistula
   E. Pneumothorax

2. **PaO$_2$:**
   A. Decreases at high altitude
   B. Does not change in severe anaemia
   C. Level of 13.5 kPa signifies type I respiratory failure
   D. Is always normal in right to left cardiac shunts
   E. Levels below 8 kPa suggest a need for assisted ventilation

3. **Hypocarbia is common in:**
   A. Hyperventilation
   B. Alveolar hypoventilation
   C. Sedative drugs
   D. Myasthenia gravis
   E. Type II respiratory failure

4. **General features of malignancy:**
   A. Fever                B. Cachexia
   C. Thrombotic episodes   D. Anaemia
   E. Absence of metastasis

5. **Randomised controlled trial:**
   A. Is a useful method in modern clinical research
   B. Is directed by the patient
   C. Is always retrospective
   D. May require ethical committee approval in the United Kingdom
   E. Is not recommended in surgical practice

---

1. A:T, B:T, C:F, D:T, E:T      2. A:T, B:T, C:F, D:F, E:T
3. A:T, B:F, C:F, D:F, E:F      4. A:T, B:T, C:T, D:T, E:F
5. A:T, B:F, C:F, D:T, E:F

6. **Informed consent:**
   A. Is obtained only from individuals aged 21 years or more
   B. May not be necessary in life-threatening situations in an unconscious patient
   C. Should be aimed at answering all questions with honesty
   D. Should ideally be taken from a relative of the patient
   E. Is not necessary in paediatric surgery

7. **Chemotherapy is used for:**
   A. Seminoma of testis
   B. Teratoma of testis
   C. Breast carcinoma with multiple secondaries
   D. Renal cell carcinoma, as a primary treatment
   E. Gastric carcinoma

8. **LASER in surgical practice:**
   A. Adequate eye protection should be worn
   B. Is not recommended for GI system
   C. Class 4 have a minimum risk and therefore commonly used
   D. Used for portwine stains
   E. Nd:YAG useful for some bladder tumours

9. **Ca Colon:**
   A. Risk increases with long standing ulcerative colitis
   B. Duke B denotes spread to the mesenteric lymph nodes
   C. Is associated with p53 gene mutation
   D. Is common in first degree relatives of affected patients
   E. May spread to liver and bone

---

6. A:F, B:T, C:T, D:F, E:F     7. A:T, B:T, C:T, D:F, E:T
8. A:T, B:F, C:F, D:T, E:T     9. A:T, B:F, C:T, D:T, E:T

10. Missile injuries:
    A. All wounds should be closed primarily
    B. Require tetanus prophylaxis
    C. Early thoracotomy is indicated if mediastinum is involved
    D. Wounds of the chest should be left open
    E. Involved nerves should be treated by primary nerve exploration and repair

11. Suture materials causing minimal reactions:
    A. Silk
    B. Chromic catgut
    C. Polypropylene
    D. Polyglycolic acid
    E. Polydiaxonone

12. Immunosuppressants:
    A. Cyclosporin A
    B. Prednisolone
    C. Non-steroidal anti-inflammatory drugs
    D. Erythromycin
    E. Methotrexate

13. Disseminated intravascular coagulation:
    A. Increased FDP
    B. Increased PT
    C. Common in septic shock
    D. Fibrinogen levels correlate with severity
    E. Bleeding is rarely a problem

14. Premalignant conditions of liver:
    A. Hepatitis C
    B. Hepatitis B
    C. Polycystic liver disease
    D. Haemangiomas
    E. Cirrhosis

---

10. A:F, B:T, C:T, D:F, E:F     11. A:F, B:F, C:T, D:T, E:T
12. A:T, B:T, C:F, D:F, E:T     13. A:T, B:T, C:T, D:T, E:F
14. A:T, B:T, C:F, D:F, E:T

15. **Shock:**
    A. Leads to poor tissue perfusion
    B. Has a particularly bad prognosis if the cause is cardiogenic
    C. Usually self limiting
    D. Catecholamines should be used in all cases
    E. Is hypovolemic, following trauma, in most cases

16. **Endotoxins:**
    A. Are produced by gram-negative bacteria
    B. Are non-specific and can affect all organs and tissues
    C. Are highly antigenic polypeptides
    D. Are present in the cell wall of the bacteria
    E. Causing septic shock are commonly produced by clostridia group of organisms

17. **Spleen is:**
    A. A major storage organ for platelets
    B. Is responsible for entrapment of >120 days old RBCs
    C. Involved in haemopoiesis in fetal life
    D. A site for bilirubin formation
    E. Structurally composed of white and red pulps

18. **A Type I diabetic having a major intra-abdominal surgery:**
    A. Must continue to take s/c insulin upto 30 minutes prior to surgery
    B. Requires IV infusion of dextrose on day of surgery
    C. Has an increased risk of postoperative infection
    D. Should receive IV insulin in perioperative period
    E. Needs regular monitoring of blood sugar

19. **Carbuncle is more common in:**
    A. Diabetics
    B. Back of neck
    C. Tissues with reduced vitality
    D. Axilla
    E. Palms and soles

15. A:T, B:T, C:F, D:F, E:T    16. A:T, B:T, C:F, D:T, E:F
17. A:T, B:T, C:T, D:F, E:T    18. A:F, B:T, C:T, D:T, E:T
19. A:T, B:T, C:T, D:F, E:F

20. **The risk for venous thrombosis is increased after:**
    A. Total hip replacement
    B. Administration of heparin
    C. Surgery for malignancy
    D. Hormonal replacement therapy
    E. The use of compression stockings and foot pumps in the perioperative period

21. **Early mobilisation:**
    A. Decreases the risk of thrombosis
    B. Prevents chest infection
    C. Delays wound healing
    D. Increases the chances of haemorrhage after a total knee replacement
    E. Reduces the incidences of bedsores

22. **Cholecystectomy:**
    A. Prophylactic antibiotics are indicated
    B. Informed consent should be taken
    C. Identification of Calot's triangle is important
    D. Always successful when performed laparoscopically
    E. Can lead to haemorrhage

23. **Paronychia:**
    A. Caused by careless nail trimming
    B. Characterised by swelling and tenderness of the nail fold
    C. Surgery is contraindicated
    D. MRSA is the commonest causative organism
    E. Also known as 'felon'

24. **Causes of postoperative jaundice:**
    A. Massive blood transfusion
    B. Halothane
    C. Ligation of common bile duct
    D. Chest infection
    E. Bleeding

---

20. A:T, B:F, C:T, D:T, E:F
22. A:T, B:T, C:T, D:F, E:T
24. A:T, B:T, C:T, D:T, E:F

21. A:T, B:T, C:F, D:F, E:T
23. A:T, B:T, C:F, D:F, E:F

25. **Preoperative antibiotics for colonic surgery:**
    A. Sterilises colonic mucosa
    B. Should be started 72 hours preoperative
    C. Should cover both Gm +ve and Gm −ve organisms
    D. Must be avoided in patients resistant to penicillin
    E. Should rapidly achieve tissue levels above the minimum inhibitory concentration

26. **Gas gangrene:**
    A. Is caused by clostridia
    B. Endotoxin causes tissue damage
    C. Crepitus and colour changes in the affected area are important signs
    D. May cause renal failure
    E. Hyperbaric oxygen is used in some institutions

27. **Malignant melanoma is:**
    A. Less malignant if Breslow's depth of invasion is 0.75 mm
    B. More malignant if Clark's Grade V
    C. Common in exposed parts of the body
    D. Never seen in Caucasians
    E. Associated with satellite lesions

28. **Burkitt's lymphoma:**
    A. Is common in African children
    B. Is associated with Reed-Sternberg cells
    C. May show remission with cyclophosphamide
    D. Frequently presents as tumour in the jaw
    E. On microscopy may show 'starry sky' appearance

29. **Hodgkin's lymphoma:**
    A. Subtype nodular sclerosing, is more common in males
    B. Weight loss and night sweats may be present
    C. Peak incidence is seen in early childhood
    D. Prognosis is independepent of the stage
    E. Associated with EB virus

25. A:F, B:F, C:T, D:F, E:T    26. A:T, B:F, C:T, D:T, E:T
27. A:T, B:T, C:T, D:F, E:T    28. A:T, B:F, C:T, D:T, E:T
29. A:F, B:T, C:F, D:F, E:T

30. **Ulnar nerve injury at wrist causes:**
    A. Loss of abduction of thumb
    B. Loss of abduction of middle finger
    C. Wasting of hypothenar muscles
    D. Loss of flexion of DIP joints of the fingers
    E. Loss of sensations in the medial aspect of middle finger

31. **Cervical spine injury:**
    A. Can be ruled out if no pain or neurological deficit is present
    B. Can be ruled out only by X-ray
    C. Should be suspected in an unconscious patient if there is bradycardia and a low BP
    D. Should be always suspected in patients with major maxillofacial injuries
    E. Can present without any radiological signs, in children

32. **Brainstem death:**
    A. Absence of spontaneous respiration when disconnected from a ventilator
    B. Nystagmus on caloric tests
    C. Lower limb movements on supraorbital pressure
    D. Unreactive pupils
    E. Positive corneal reflex

33. **Tension pneumothorax causes:**
    A. Increased air entry         B. Decreased resonance
    C. Cyanosis                    D. Shift of mediastinum
    E. Paradoxical respiration

34. **The diaphragm:**
    A. Transmits the aorta at the level of the tenth thoracic vertebra
    B. Receives its motor supply from the phrenic nerves (Root value C3-5)
    C. Is pierced by the oesophagus at T12
    D. Opening for the vena cava is located at L2
    E. Is supplied by the lower five intercostals nerves

30. A:F, B:T, C:T, D:F, E:F        31. A:F, B:F, C:T, D:T, E:T
32. A:T, B:F, C:F, D:T, E:F        33. A:F, B:F, C:T, D:T, E:F
34. A:F, B:T, C:F, D:F, E:T

35. **Warfarin:**
    A. Is indicated for prophylaxis in atrial fibrillation
    B. Dose should be increased preoperatively in the joint replacement surgery
    C. Is contraindicated in established cases of DVT
    D. Effects may be reversed by the administration of intravenous vitamin K
    E. Reduces the concentration of vitamin A dependent factors

36. **Causes of hypercalcaemia:**
    A. Secondaries       B. Hypoparathyroidism
    C. Sarcoidosis       D. Hypervitaminosis D
    E. Lithium intake

37. **Compartment syndrome:**
    A. Is associated with ischaemia
    B. Excessive pain on passive stretching the muscles is a consistent finding
    C. Is never seen in the thigh
    D. May cause Volkmann's ischaemic contracture
    E. Ultrasound is diagnostic and indicated in all cases

38. **Postoperative atelectasis:**
    A. Is a common complication after surgery
    B. Antibiotics are usually not necessary
    C. Is more common in patients with COPD
    D. Chest physiotherapy is useful in treatment
    E. May delay mobilisation in a patient who has undergone THR

39. **Aortic rupture is associated with:**
    A. Increased superior mediastinal shadow in chest X-ray (PA view)
    B. Radiofemoral delay
    C. Hoarseness of voice
    D. Paradoxical respiration
    E. Deceleration injuries

---

35. A:T, B:F, C:F, D:T, E:F       36. A:T, B:F, C:T, D:T, E:T
37. A:T, B:T, C:F, D:T, E:F       38. A:T, B:F, C:T, D:T, E:T
39. A:T, B:T, C:T, D:F, E:T

40. **Myocardial pre-load:**
    A. Decreased, in venous constriction
    B. Decreased, in head down position
    C. A fall, causes a rise in end-diastolic volume
    D. A rise, casues a fall in stroke volume
    E. Does not influence cardiac output

41. **Fat emboli:**
    A. Can be prevented by adequate oxygen and fluid resuscitation
    B. May be increased by immobilisation of fractures
    C. Produce a characteristic petechial rash
    D. Are generated while reaming a fractured bone
    E. Can be diagnosed with reasonable accuracy by performing a V/Q scan

42. **Coagulation abnormalities are associated with:**
    A. Postoperative wound infection
    B. Liver disease
    C. DIC
    D. Warfarin intake
    E. Protein C and S deficiency

43. **Breast carcinoma commonly metastases to:**
    A. Liver
    B. Lung
    C. Bone
    D. Spleen
    E. Contralateral breast

44. **Screening programmes in the United Kingdom:**
    A. Malignant melanoma
    B. Cervical cancer
    C. Fracture neck of femur
    D. Back pain
    E. Breast cancer

40. A:T, B:F, C:F, D:F, E:F        41. A:T, B:F, C:T, D:T, E:F
42. A:F, B:T, C:T, D:T, E:T        43. A:T, B:T, C:T, D:F, E:F
44. A:F, B:T, C:F, D:F, E:T

45. **Hyperthermia:**
    A. Is defined as a core temperature above 38°C
    B. Is seen following the use of certain inhalational anaesthetic agents
    C. Involves resetting of the hypothalamic thermostat
    D. Due to suxamethonium, may be reversed by dantrolene
    E. Usually causes alkalosis

46. **Hernia operation is not recommended as a day case procedure in the following situations:**
    A. Requirement of general anaesthetic
    B. BMI > 35
    C. No responsible adult available at home
    D. MI 2 weeks ago
    E. Patients on Warfarin

47. **Features of strangulated hernia:**
    A. Sudden pain over the hernia followed by generalised colicky pain
    B. Pink bowel with normal peristalsis
    C. More common in inguinal than femoral hernias
    D. Close observation followed by elective repair is recommended
    E. Expansile cough is a diagnostic sign

48. **Wound healing involves:**
    A. Activation of osteoclasts as a primary event
    B. Langerhan's giant cells
    C. Contraction
    D. Reorientation of collagen fibrils
    E. Vasodilatation and edema

---

45. A:F, B:T, C:T, D:T, E:F       46. A:F, B:T, C:T, D:T, E:T
47. A:T, B:F, C:F, D:F, E:F       48. A:F, B:F, C:T, D:T, E:T

49. **Tourniquet:**
    A. Can be used for about three and a half hours in the lower limb
    B. Pressure in the cuff should be approximately equal to one-third of diastolic pressure
    C. Pressures (max) for upper and lower limbs are roughly the same
    D. Is contraindicated in carpal tunnel decompression
    E. Provides haemostasis and makes surgery easier

50. **Smoking is associated with:**
    A. Malignant melanoma     B. Ca urinary bladder
    C. Burkitt's tumour     D. Ca larynx
    E. Wilms' tumour

51. **Lignocaine:**
    A. Maximum safe dose is 150 mg as plain solution
    B. Is cardiotoxic
    C. Blocks pathways involved in the formation of inflammatory agents
    D. Also provides prolonged sedation when administered locally
    E. Should never be used for procedures on fingers

52. **A fracture neck of humerus may cause:**
    A. Wrist drop
    B. Deltoid paralysis
    C. Loss of power in interossei
    D. Paralysis of Abductor pollicis brevis
    E. Sensory loss in the area overlying deltoid

53. **Achalasia:**
    A. Occurs due to abundance of ganglionic cells in myeneteric plexus
    B. Has no association with malignancy
    C. Is treated with Heller's myotomy
    D. Is characterised by a typical 'bird's beak' appearance on barium studies
    E. Is characterised by very low resting pressures of lower oesophageal sphincter

49. A:F, B:F, C:F, D:F, E:T     50. A:F, B:T, C:F, D:T, E:F
51. A:T, B:T, C:F, D:F, E:F     52. A:F, B:T, C:F, D:F, E:T
53. A:F, B:F, C:T, D:T, E:F

54. **Mesothelioma:**
    A. Chest X-ray is used for definitive diagnosis
    B. Dyspnoea and chest pain are common
    C. Exposure to asbestos is a risk factor
    D. Very good prognosis with a median survival of 8-10 years
    E. Involvement of peritoneum and pericardium has been reported

55. **Postoperative complications:**

| | |
|---|---|
| A. A temperature of 38.7, 5 days following cholecystectomy, with induration and tenderness over the wound and neutrophilia. | 1. Myocardial infarction<br>2. Pulmonary embolism |
| B. A 68-year-old patient on aspirin has brief loss of consciousness and paraperesis 12 hours after a dynamic hip screw fixation | 3. Acute renal failure<br>4. Atelectesis<br>5. Stroke |
| C. An 80 years old patient with IHD develops chest pain, cough and a WCC of 22.6 thirty-six hours after operation. ABGs and ECG are normal | 6. Wound |
| D. A 73 years old female with postoperative swelling in the operated leg after a TKR complains of severe right sided chest pain and shortness of breath | |
| E. A 76-year-old man on aspirin develops confusion and drowsiness 12 hours following surgery for a bleeding tumour. Post-operative potassium is 6.2 | |

54. A:F, B:T, C:T, D:F, E:T    55. A:6, B:5, C:4, D:2, E:3

56. **Microorganisms:**
    A. A surgeon is not allowed to carry out any invasive procedures throughout his life after a recent blood test even though he was HIV negative
    B. Severe pain and vesicular eruptions in the chest
    C. A young adult with lymphadenopathy, fever and Kaposi' sarcoma
    D. Jaundice following a blood transfusion few months ago. The patient is core antigen positive
    E. Nasopharyngeal carcinoma

    1. Coxsackie A virus
    2. HIV
    3. Papilloma viruses
    4. Epstein Barr viruses
    5. Herpes zoster virus
    6. Hepatitis B virus
    7. Hepatitis A virus

57. **Drugs in surgery:**
    A. Severe nausea and vomiting after chemotherapy
    B. Adjuvant therapy following wide local excision of a breast tumour in a postmenopausal female
    C. Known to be effective against Duke C tumour
    D. Dihydrofolate reductase inhibitor
    E. Alkylating anti-cancer agent

    1. Adriamycin
    2. Cyclophosphamide
    3. Busulphan
    4. Methotrexate
    5. Tamoxifen
    6. Fluorouracil
    7. Ondansetron
    8. Nifedipine

58. A patient develops respiratory distress. He is known to use inhalers for many years. Arterial blood gas analysis shows:

| | |
|---|---|
| pH | 7.30 |
| PCO$_2$ | 8.9 |
| PO$_2$ | 7.31 |
| HCO$_3^-$ | 38.6 |
| BE | +7.4 |
| SBE | +7.9 |
| Oxygen saturation | 82% |

**Which of the following statements are true about metabolic abnormalities in this patient:**
A. Respiratory acidosis
B. Compensated metabolic alkalosis
C. Compensated respiratory alkalosis
D. Primary metabolic acidosis
E. Normal blood gas result for a patient with long-standing COPD

59. **Features of oesophageal varices:**
    A. Suggestive of pulmonary hypertension
    B. Often respond to sclerosant therapy
    C. Important cause of upper GI haemorrhage
    D. Caput medusae
    E. Splenomegaly

60. **Complications of total parenteral nutrition:**
    A. Hyperglycaemia
    B. Hypoglycaemia
    C. Infection
    D. Metabolic acidosis
    E. Fatty liver

58. A:T, B:T, C:F, D:F, E:F     59. A:F, B:T, C:T, D:T, E:T
60. A:T, B:T, C:T, D:T, E:T

## PAPER II

*(Answer the following questions as True or False; Time Allowed:120 minutes)*

1. **Breast Screening Programme in the UK:**
   A. Includes all women in the 25-45 age group
   B. Aims at identifying advanced cases of breast cancer
   C. Has proved to be unsuccessful and is likely to be abolished soon
   D. Involves mammography
   E. Has led to overdiagnosis of DCIS in certain cases

2. **Postoperative pyrexia:**
   A. Within 48 hours is strongly suggestive of a wound infection
   B. After 3 weeks indicates pulmonary embolism
   C. Within 6 hours needs aggressive antibiotic therapy
   D. At 36 hours should be treated by high doses of heparin
   E. Within the first 24 hours is due to increase in the basal metabolic rate

3. **Morphine:**
   A. Primarily acts on Kappa receptors
   B. Causes meiosis and constipation
   C. Is safe to use in respiratory depression
   D. Is known to cause delayed gastric emptying
   E. Subcutaneous administration is contraindicated

4. **Following are important features of hypovolemic shock:**
   A. Tachycardia
   B. Increased urine output
   C. Hypoxia
   D. Hypotension
   E. Cold extremeties

---

1. A:F, B:F, C:F, D:T, E:T      2. A:F, B:F, C:F, D:F, E:T
3. A:F, B:T, C:F, D:T, E:F      4. A:T, B:F, C:T, D:T, E:T

5. **Vicryl:**
   A. Is a non-absorbable suture
   B. Commonly used in vascular anastomosis
   C. Is obtained from intestinal mucosa
   D. Loses all its strength after 5 days
   E. Is widely used in orthopaedic surgery

6. **Fine needle aspiration cytology:**
   A. Has no role in thyroid swellings
   B. For neck lumps usually requires a general anaesthetic
   C. Is not recommended for breast lumps
   D. Has a poor sensitivity even with good technique
   E. May be performed under imaging

7. **Fluid:**
   A. Average normal daily loss in urine is about 3.5 litres
   B. About 12 litres is present as plasma in the body
   C. Retention may cause hyponatremia
   D. Average normal amount in expired air is about 400 ml/day
   E. Normal adult daily requirement is 2-3 litres

8. **Secondaries in the bone usually metastasis from:**
   A. Breast              B. Bronchus
   C. Kidney             D. Thyroid
   E. Prostate

9. **Acute renal failure:**
   A. In postoperative patients is most commonly due to post-renal causes
   B. May necessitate CVP and pulmonary artery floatation catheter monitoring
   C. Is common in severe sepsis
   D. May lead to a potentially life-threatening hyperkalaemia
   E. In postoperative patients may be managed by rapid correction of dehydration

5. A:F, B:F, C:F, D:F, E:T       6. A:F, B:F, C:F, D:F, E:T
7. A:F, B:F, C:T, D:F, E:T       8. A:T, B:T, C:T, D:T, E:T
9. A:F, B:T, C:F, D:T, E:T

10. **In DIC:**
    A. Sepsis is an important causative factor
    B. PT and PTT are markedly reduced
    C. Fibrinogen levels are typically low
    D. Thrombocytopenia is a common feature
    E. Thrombin activation is the key event

11. **Oxygen dissociation curve:**
    A. Shifts to the right with a rise in temperature
    B. Shifts to the left with a fall in the levels of 2,3- DPG
    C. Is not affected by any change in $PCO_2$
    D. Is a plot of percent saturation of Hb as a function of $PCO_2$
    E. Has a sigmoid shape

12. **A 35 years old man is rescued several hours from a collapsed house. His left leg was found sandwiched between two concrete blocks. On examination, he is fully conscious, has an intact airway and normal breathing and circulation. Crepitus is felt over the calf muscles, and the overlying skin is discoloured. Besides few lacerations on the lower limbs, there are no other obvious injuries. He is airlifted to a district hospital and the radiograph of the chest does not reveal any injury. X-ray of the leg also shows no bony injury. Subsequently, he becomes confused, hypotensive and oliguric.:**
    A. His leg needs to be immobilized urgently in a plaster cast
    B. Full skeletal survey to rule out any major fracture is a top priority
    C. Oxygen and fluid resuscitation is indicated
    D. Gas may be present in the radiograph of the leg
    E. Early surgery is indicated

---

10. A:T, B:F, C:T, D:T, E:T        11.  A:T, B:T, C:F, D:F, E:T
12. A:F, B:F, C:T, D:T, E:T

13. A 52-year-old lorry driver develops a penetrating injury to the abdomen following an accident. He develops a splenic rupture and other injuries which are successfully dealt with, at a district hospital. 48 hours after surgery, he develops a high temperature, a significant fall in the blood pressure (80/50mmHg) and an increased repiratory rate 24/min. The abdominal wound shows some discharge and signs of inflammation. His peripheries are warm and urine output is falling:
    A. The most likely cause is sepsis
    B. Operative intervention may be necessary
    C. Adequate resuscitation and monitoring is recommended
    D. S. Amylase estimation is urgently required
    E. Antibiotic therapy should be commenced after the blood culture results are available

14. Diabetes insipidus causes:
    A. A rise in in the extracellular fluid osmolality
    B. A fall in the intracellular osmolality
    C. Depletion of extracellular but not intracellular fluid volume
    D. The daily urinary volume to increase to a maximum of 2.5 litres per day
    E. Excretion of urine with a persistently low osmolality

15. Acidosis can cause:
    A. Enhanced secretion of potassium by renal tubules
    B. Hyperventilaion
    C. A drop in the pH
    D. Renal failure
    E. Tetany

16. Initial response to haemorrhage:
    A. Tachycardia
    B. Increased cardiac contractility
    C. Marked reduction in angiotensin and ADH levels
    D. Elevation of circulating epinephrine levels
    E. Rise in aldosterone levels

---

13. A:T, B:T, C:T, D:F, E:F          14. A:T, B:F, C:F, D:F, E:T
15. A:F, B:T, C:T, D:T, E:F          16. A:T, B:T, C:F, D:T, E:T

17. **Tumour markers are used for:**
    A. Establishing a definitive diagnosis
    B. Screening
    C. Prognosis
    D. Detecting recurrence
    E. Monitoring

18. **Acute phase reactants:**
    A. Most common site of synthesis is spleen
    B. Raised in infections and following surgery
    C. Viral in origin
    D. Fibrinogen is an example
    E. Proteinaceous in nature

19. **Tumour necrosis factor-alpha:**
    A. May cause multiple organ dysfunction syndrome
    B. Induces fever
    C. Is also known as cachectin
    D. Is predominantly anti-inflammatory
    E. Causes fibroblast proliferation

20. **Axillary node dissection for Ca breast results in:**
    A. Frozen shoulder
    B. Lymphoedema
    C. Numbness down the inner side of the arm
    D. Spread to the contralateral side
    E. Determination of prognosis and treatment

21. **Horner's syndrome is characterised by:**
    A. Mydriasis
    B. Anhidrosis
    C. Enophthalmos
    D. Ptosis
    E. Loss of sympathetic tone

---

17. A:F, B:T, C:T, D:T, E:T    18. A:F, B:T, C:F, D:T, E:T
19. A:T, B:T, C:T, D:F, E:T    20. A:T, B:T, C:T, D:F, E:T
21. A:F, B:T, C:T, D:T, E:T

22. **Compartment syndrome:**
    A. Repurfusion injury is an established cause
    B. Loss of peripheral pulses is an early sign
    C. Motor weakness suggests bad prognosis
    D. Can be easily misdiagnosed as DVT
    E. Urgent fasciotomy is indicated if there is no improvement

23. **Features of carpal tunnel syndrome:**
    A. Seen in pregnancy and Rheumatoid arthritis
    B. Phalen's test is useful for diagnosis
    C. Wasting of hypothenar muscles
    D. Absence of sensations over thenar eminence
    E. Steroid injection causes resolution of symptoms in 93% cases

24. **Magnesium:**
    A. Absorbtion takes place in distal collecting segment only
    B. Competes with calcium for resorption
    C. Deficiency causes arrythmias
    D. Excess causes tetany and paraesthesia
    E. Levels should be monitored in TPN

25. **Ca oesophagus:**
    A. More than 50% occur in proximal one-third
    B. Radiotherapy is often used in unfit patients
    C. Involvement of coeliac nodes suggest only local spread and therefore good prognosis
    D. 5 years survival is only 5-10 percent
    E. Endoscopic ultrasound is a reliable method for staging

26. **Cushing's response in head injury consists includes:**
    A. Reduced respiratory rate
    B. Increased heart rate
    C. Increased systolic blood pressure
    D. Fall in pulse pressure
    E. Decrease in total peripheral resistance

---

22. A:T, B:F, C:T, D:T, E:T      23. A:T, B:T, C:F, D:F, E:F
24. A:F, B:T, C:T, D:F, E:T      25. A:F, B:T, C:F, D:T, E:T
26. A:T, B:F, C:T, D:F, E:F

27. **Ethylene oxide:**
    A. Is useful for heat sensitive equipment
    B. Most commonly used method for sterilising syringes and catheters
    C. Has a weak bactericidal activity
    D. Is carcinogenic
    E. Has very low penetration

28. **Liver disease may lead to:**
    A. Pulmonary edema
    B. Hepatorenal syndrome
    C. Prolonged prothrombin time
    D. Increase in serum albumin
    E. Wound infection

29. **Complications of fractures:**
    A. Volkmann's ischemic contracture
    B. Myositis ossificans
    C. Fat embolism
    D. Carpal tunnel syndrome
    E. Crush syndrome

30. **Lung volumes and capacities:**
    A. Normal tidal volume is 1.5 litres
    B. Residual volume is the volume of gas remaining in lungs after maximum inspiration
    C. Functional residual capacity is the sum of ERV and RV
    D. Volume in anatomical dead space is about 150 ml
    E. Normal $FEV_1/FVC = 0.8$

31. **For surgery on large bowel, the following are important:**
    A. Bowel preparation by oral purgatives
    B. Prophylactic antibiotics at the time of surgery
    C. Informed consent
    D. Tourniquet
    E. IV fluids started 48 hours preoperative in all cases

---

27. A:T, B:F, C:F, D:T, E:F      28. A:T, B:T, C:T, D:F, E:T
29. A:T, B:T, C:T, D:T, E:T      30. A:F, B:F, C:T, D:T, E:T
31. A:T, B:T, C:T, D:F, E:F

32. **Pro-inflammatory cytokines:**
    A. Interleukin-1
    B. Interleukin-8
    C. Interleukin-13
    D. Transforming growth factor-β
    E. Interleukin-4

33. **Features of anaemia include:**
    A. Reduced blood viscosity
    B. Reduced cardiac output
    C. Increased heart rate
    D. Reduced peripheral resistance
    E. Reduced $O_2$ delivery

34. **Effects of positive pressure ventilation:**
    A. Peripheral vasodilatation    B. Sodium retention
    C. Decreased compliance    D. Reduced BP
    E. Barotrauma

35. **Obesity:**
    A. Reduces the risk of infection
    B. Causes an increased risk of aspiration pneumonitis after GA
    C. Is a limiting factor for day care surgery
    D. Enhances gastric emptying
    E. Increases the intra-abdominal pressure

36. **Massive blood transfusion**
    A. Causes acute respiratory distress syndrome
    B. Is defined as transfusion of a volume of blood greater than the recipient's blood volume in less than 24 hours
    C. Hypothermia and hyperkalaemia are known complications
    D. Alkalosis is very common esp. in severe renal disease
    E. Rapid infusion of IV gluconate is recommended

---

32. A:T, B:T, C:F, D:F, E:F    33. A:F, B:F, C:T, D:F, E:T
34. A:F, B:T, C:T, D:T, E:T    35. A:F, B:T, C:T, D:F, E:T
36. A:T, B:T, C:T, D:F, E:F

37. **Features of pulmonary embolism:**
    A. Raised BP
    B. Pleuritic chest pain is the earliest symptom
    C. Dyspnoea is the commonest symptom
    D. Respiratory alkalosis
    E. Mismatch on V/Q scan

38. **Sickle cell disease:**
    A. Autosomal recessive
    B. Valine substitution for glutamine in Hb chain
    C. Oxygen and fluid administration -important in the perioperative period
    D. Use of tourniquet recommended to avoid bleeding
    E. Electrophoresis useful for diagnosis

39. **The following tumours are markedly radiosensitive:**
    A. Ca stomach
    B. Malignant melanoma
    C. Hypernephroma
    D. Medulloblastomas
    E. Squamous cell carcinoma of the skin

40. **For methicillin resistant *Staphylococcus aureus* (MRSA) infections, the following approach may be adopted:**
    A. Isolation of all contacts
    B. Isolation of all patients having MRSA infections
    C. Random screening of health care workers
    D. Antibiotics to all groups—patient, carrier and health care workers
    E. No action necessary

41. ***H. pylori:***
    A. Is gram-negative
    B. Can be identified by histology and urea breath test
    C. Is associated with gastric cancer
    D. Eradication is possible by triple therapy
    E. Causes stimulation of G-cells

---

37. A:F, B:F, C:T, D:T, E:T        38.  A:F, B:T, C:T, D:T, E:T
39. A:F, B:F, C:F, D:T, E:T        40.  A:F, B:T, C:F, D:F, E:F
41. A:F, B:T,C:T, D:T, E:T

42. **Normal wound healing involves:**
    A. Osteoblast proliferation
    B. Fibroblast proliferation
    C. Angiogenesis
    D. Mediators PDGF and IL-1
    E. Inflammation

43. **Keloid scars:**
    A. Are commonly seen over the flexor surfaces
    B. Frequently outgrow the wound area
    C. Resolve spontaneously
    D. May respond to interstitial radiotherapy
    E. Are best treated with pressure or massage

44. **Fluid retention is common in:**
    A. Congestive heart failure
    B. Anorexia nervosa
    C. Diabetes insipidus
    D. Cushing's disease
    E. Cirrhosis

45. **Loop diuretics:**
    A. Act on thick ascending loop of Henle
    B. Severe hyperkalaemia is the most common complication
    C. Are contraindicated in renal failure with anuria
    D. Common example is triamterene
    E. May cause hyponatremia and hypomagnesemia

46. ***Staphylococcus aureus* is the commonest causative organism in the following:**
    A. Toxic shock syndrome
    B. Osteomyelitis in a 3-year-old-girl
    C. Necrotising fascitis
    D. Vincent's angina
    E. Gas gangrene

---

42. A:F, B:T, C:T, D:T, E:T
44. A:T, B:F, C:F, D:T, E:T
46. A:T, B:F, C:F, D:F, E:F
43. A:F, B:T, C:F, D:T, E:F
45. A:T, B:F, C:T, D:F, E:T

47. Following are the adverse effects of tamoxifen:
    A. Endometrial hyperplasia
    B. Vaginal discharge
    C. MI
    D. Thrombosis
    E. Hot flushes

48. The following are the nerve roots for:
    A. Anal reflex S1
    B. Diaphragm C3, 4, 5
    C. Knee jerk L3, 4
    D. Shoulder abductor C7
    E. Hip flexion L2, 3

49. Opportunistic infection is associated with:
    A. Anti-inflammatories
    B. AIDS
    C. Steroid use
    D. Organ transplantation
    E. Chemotherapy

50. Diclofenac:
    A. Is a selective cycloxigenase-2 inhibitor
    B. Decreases platelet aggregation
    C. Given chronically may cause interstitial nephritis
    D. May be given IV
    E. Causes gastric ulcers

51. Following are the predisposing factors for Ca colon:
    A. Familial polyposis coli
    B. Diverticulitis
    C. Crohn's disease
    D. Ulcerative colitis
    E. Proctalgia fugax

47. A:T, B:T, C:F, D:T, E:T        48. A:F, B:T, C:T, D:F, E:T
49. A:F, B:T, C:T, D:T, E:T        50. A:F, B:T, C:T, D:T, E:T
51. A:T, B:F, C:T, D:T, E:F

52. **Shock:**
    - **A.** Early treatment by catecholamines is indicated
    - **B.** Baroreceptor response stimulates the sympathetic nervous system
    - **C.** A systolic blood pressure of 100 mmHg, pulse rate of 96 following a loss of 1350 ml of blood corresponds with Class III shock
    - **D.** May be caused by pneumothorax
    - **E.** 3:1 rule is used for fluid replacement

53. **Melanoma:**
    - **A.** Breslow's classification indicates the depth of involvement
    - **B.** Breslow's thickness of 0.75 mm indicates good prognosis
    - **C.** Clark's grade III indicates subcutaneous involvement
    - **D.** Subungual melanoma is a type of acral lentiginous melanoma
    - **E.** Nodular melanoma is the least malignant type

54. **Following is true about Ultrasound:**
    - **A.** High electromagnetic waves are generated during screening
    - **B.** It is a first line investigation in hepatobiliary disease
    - **C.** Intraluminal examination of vessels, vagina and rectum is possible
    - **D.** Radiation is a frequent problem
    - **E.** Not recommended for cystic swellings

55. **A pelvic abscess:**
    - **A.** Vulval edema is a established sign
    - **B.** Constipation is the commonest symptom
    - **C.** Per rectal mucous discharge after peritonitis is an important sign
    - **D.** Frequently requires urgent laparotomy
    - **E.** Common sequel of anastomic leakage following large bowel and rectal surgery

---

52. A:F, B:T, C:F, D:T, E:T     53. A:T, B:T, C:F, D:T, E:F
54. A:F, B:T, C:T, D:F, E:F     55. A:T, B:F, C:T, D:F, E:T

## 56. Peripheral nerve lesions

A. Painless weakness of finger extension without any associated wrist drop

B. Wasting of thenar eminence, paraesthesia of the radial three and a half digits, but no palmar sensory loss and no weakness of flexion of fingers or thumb

C. Wrist drop and sensory loss in posterior aspect of arm and forearm and autonomous zone after sleeping awkwardly in a chair

D. Weakness of interossei and sensory disturbance in the medial one and a half digits after ulnar head resection in a rheumatoid patient

E. Loss of abduction and sensations over 'regimental badge' area after a humeral fracture

1. Radial nerve injury at wrist
2. Median nerve lesion at the wrist
3. Ulnar nerve injury at the wrist
4. Radial nerve injury in the axilla
5. Posterior interosseus nerve injury
6. Radial nerve injury in the arm
7. Musculocutaneous nerve injury in the arm
8. Axillary nerve injury in the shoulder

56. A:5, B: 2, C:4, D:3, E:8

57. **Tumour markers:**
    A. Elevated in 44% cases of Dukes' grade C and about 65% patients with distant metastasis in colorectal cancer
    B. Raised in hepatocellular carcinoma, cirrhosis and hepatitis
    C. High levels seen in pregnancy, teratomas and hydatidiform mole
    D. Elevated in more than 95% cases of advanced ovarian cancer.May also be elevated in I trimester of pregnancy, cirrhosis with ascites and endometriosis
    E. High levels detected in advanced prostatic cancer and also in some cases with BPH

1. Ca 15-3
2. PSA
3. hCG
4. Alpha fetoprotein
5. Ca 19-9
6. CEA
7. Ca 125
8. Ca 72-4

57. A:6, B:4, C:3, D:7, E:2

58. **Investigations:**
    A. A haemodynamically stable patient with a suspected blunt trauma to the abdomen
    B. Uncontrolled Crohn's disease with multiple discharging perianal sinuses
    C. A patient with prostate carcinoma complaining of pain in the back and chest wall
    D. First line investigation in a postoperative patient with constipation, vomiting and abdominal distension
    E. 35-year-old patient with sudden onset of back pain after heavy weight lifting with motor weakness, perineal anesthesia and urinary retention

1. Ultrasound
2. MRI scan
3. CT scan
4. X-ray abdomen
5. Bone scan
6. Mammography
7. IVP
8. Open biopsy

58. A:3, B:2, C:5, D:4, E:2

## 59. Metabolic derangement:

A. Tall tented T waves, widened QRS complexes on ECG with arrythmias after acute renal failure

B. Severe abdominal pain, constipation, polyuria, confusion, bone pains and renal stones

C. Muscle weakness, hypotonia, raised bicarbonate and ECG changes after prolonged treatment with a loop diuretic

D. Confusion, seizures, anorexia, with SIADH

E. Tetany, carpopedal spasm and ECG changes after thyroid surgery

1. Hypervitaminosis D
2. Hyperkalaemia
3. Hypokalaemia
4. Hyponatraemia
5. Hypocalcaemia
6. Hypercalcaemia
7. Hyponatraemia
8. Hypernatraemia

59. A:2, B:6, C:3, D:7, E:5

60. **Liver diseases:**
    A. 30-year-old IV drug abuser with hepatomegaly, jaundice and positive surface antigen. He had normal serology 8 weeks ago
    B. Ascites, tremors, gynaecomastia and a shrunken liver in an alcoholic. No evidence of malignancy
    C. Abdominal discomfort and ascites in a young female associated with portal hypertension. Hepatic venography demonstrates occlusion of hepatic veins
    D. Hepatomegaly with ascites and dyspnoea few months after surgery for a Dukes' C colonic cancer
    E. A 38-year-old farmer has upper abdominal discomfort. Ultrasound and CT examination shows a multiloculated cyst with a floating membrane. He shows a good response with a course of albendazole.

1. Hepatitis B
2. Hepatitis A
3. Hepatocellular carcinoma
4. Hydatid liver disease
5. Budd-Chiari syndrome
6. Hemangiomas
7. Secondary deposits in liver
8. Cirrhosis of liver

---

60. A:1 /, B:8, C:5, D:7, E:4

# READER SUGGESTIONS SHEET

*Please help us to improve the quality of our publications by completing and returning this sheet to us.*

Title/Author: **MCQs for the MRCS Examination**          *by Rahij Anwar*

Your name and address:

Phone and Fax:

e-mail address:

How did you hear about this book? [please tick appropriate box (es)]

☐ Direct mail from publisher     ☐ Conference          ☐ Bookshop

☐ Book review                    ☐ Lecturer recommendation   ☐ Friends

☐ Other (please specify)         ☐ Website

Type of purchase:     ☐ Direct purchase     ☐ Bookshop     ☐ Friends

Do you have any brief comments on the book?

**Please return this sheet to the name and address given below.**

## JAYPEE BROTHERS
### MEDICAL PUBLISHERS (P) LTD
EMCA House, 23/23B Ansari Road, Daryaganj
New Delhi 110 002, India